BREATHE

Dr. Paulette D. Hubbert

Breathe

Copyright © 2018 Paulette D. Hubbert

Inspired Wholeness LLC

ISBN 978-0-9793091-2-0

LCCN 2018905369

Dedication

To my Ride or Die

About the Author

Dr. Paulette Hubbert is a native of Kansas City, Mo. She received her doctorate from Howard University and her MSW from the University of Missouri at Kansas City. As an LCSW and retired Marine she has more than 30 years of experience working with diverse groups in clinical, military, and educational environments. Her experience includes providing therapeutic and victim assistant services. Additionally, she develops and conducts seminars, trainings and workshops in the aforementioned areas. Her training and outreach activities extend to federal, state and local organizations throughout the world promoting, educating, and building awareness about the vital elements of trauma-informed doctrine, victim services and mental health.

Table of Contents

Taking a breath is the very first thing we do when we are born and the very last thing we do when we die. The very essence of our being is our breath, without it we become extinct. Remember to Breathe.

Chapter 1

"For breath is life, and if you breathe well, you will live long on the earth."
~Sanskrit proverb~

Oh no! It's happening again, I can't catch my breath, my airway is closing! I can't…my lungs are screaming for air, but I can't…I can't scream. I can feel the tightness in my throat, the crushing…. Someone, please help! (Coughing) I don't want this to be the end, not like this. I can feel the hands around my neck, the tears running down my face. I'm losing consciousness, wanting to scream, but can't, needing to run, but nowhere to go. Fight Neecy, fight the urge to take your last breath. Fight until there is no more fight. FIGHT!

"Monica, it happened again. The dream seems so real. I can still feel the sensation of the hands around my neck."

"Neecy, it is 2 am."

"You sound irritated."

"I *am* irritated! Where is Jasper?"

"He's here, sleeping like a baby."

"And as always, Jasper didn't hear you, right?"

"I don't know…I didn't ask him."

"Neecy, we keep having the same conversation. It's strange to me how you only have those dreams when Jasper spends the night, but he never hears a thing. Then, you don't wake him. Instead you call me. This has been going on for months, and I'm tired of losing sleep. Call the number I gave you."

"I can't Monica. My mother would never forgive me, and besides, it's just a dream."

"Just a dream? You call me almost every night after you wake up from a cold sweat, dreaming about being strangled, and it's just a dream?"

"I know, I know, but at least this time I didn't wake up screaming, and my bed isn't drenched with sweat like it usually is. That's a start, right?"

"Wrong Neecy. Did you do the breathing exercise I taught you? If we are not mentally healthy, we can become physically ill."

"No, I can't remember what to do."

"Do you want to do it now?"

"Yes, can we?" Ok, are you sitting comfortably?

"Yes, I'm ready."

"This breathing technique is an ancient Indian practice that involves the manipulation of breath with 3 phases–inhalation, retention and exhalation. Sit with your back straight. Place the tip of your tongue against the ridge of tissue just behind your upper front teeth and keep it there through the entire exercise. You will be exhaling through your mouth around your tongue. Exhale completely through your mouth, making a "whoosh" sound.

- Close your mouth and inhale quietly through your nose mentally count to **four**.

- Hold your breath for a count of **seven**.

- Exhale completely through your mouth, making a "whoosh" sound to a count of **eight**.

- This is one breath. Now inhale again and repeat the cycle three more times for a total of four breaths.

"Inhale quietly through your nose and exhale audibly through your mouth. The tip of your tongue stays in position the whole time. Exhalation takes twice as long as inhalation. The absolute time you spend on each phase is not important, the ratio of 4:7:8 is important. If you have trouble holding your breath, speed the exercise up but keep to the ratio of 4:7:8 for the three phases. With practice, you can things down and get used to inhaling and exhaling more and more deeply. Are you starting to feel relaxed?"

"Yes Monica, thank you."

"I have to get up early. Are we still on for lunch tomorrow?"

"Yes of course."

"Ok, I'm going to say goodnight, and tell you again to call the number I gave you. See you tomorrow."

Hmph, I don't care what Monica says, I AM getting better. I was able to wake myself this time before I broke out in a sweat and stopped breathing. That's progress, and the breathing exercise helped. Besides, what does she know? She's taken a few psychology courses and she thinks she's got me all figured out. I'll figure this out myself, but for now let me go back to bed before Jasper realizes I'm not there. His jealousy can get the best of him sometimes. If he hears me on the phone, we will be up the rest of the night arguing.

I can't believe how unreasonable he can be sometimes. It's completely normal for an emergency room doctor to get phone calls in the middle of the night. I still haven't figured out how he manages to work but call me all day. I mean, I check in with him twice a day, and it still doesn't seem to be enough to satisfy his jealousy. Either way, I'll give my dreams more thought later. There must be a reasonable explanation for all of this. Whew, Jasper is still sleeping like a baby, he doesn't know I ever left the bed.

I still can't sleep, but I dare not get up again and take a chance of waking Jasper. When he can't account for my every minute away from him, he goes ballistic. He's even gone as far as telling me he won't let me live without him. Whatever…I don't take him seriously, although Monica thinks I should. He's just talking…just his way of showing how much he loves me.

I can remember when I met Jasper. The first time I saw him I thought to myself how striking his appearance was. His dark skin and his hazel brown eyes were mesmerizing. I'm not usually attracted to a man with a beard, but his accentuates his face, and he obviously works out. His muscles were bulging through his shirt. When I saw him, I kept hoping he would notice me and to my good fortune he did.

I was leaving the hospital after a 12-hour shift. It was a beautiful day, the sun was shining brightly, the flowers were in bloom, and I remember hearing I the sound of water cascading from the large fountain in front of the hospital." Jasper was sitting on a bench by the water fountain with a cup of coffee.

I thought he was so sweet, because he had an extra cup of coffee for me. He never said who he was visiting, or why he was at the hospital, but it didn't matter, I instantly fell for him. We exchanged numbers and would spend all night talking. No matter how long my shifts were, he would be waiting for me with a hot cup of coffee when it was time to go home.

We have been inseparable since that day by the fountain. That's why I don't understand how extremely jealous he becomes when I'm out of his sight or I don't answer his phone calls right away. I would never be unfaithful to Jasper. I just can't seem to get him to understand. Besides, between work, spending time with him, and checking on my mother, I don't have time for anyone else.

Monica often complains that we don't hang out anymore. I keep explaining to her how my time is divided, but she is my ride or die, and our sisterhood bond will never be broken. I keep promising her that we are going to get back to us and I know I need to make good on that promise, but I'm so busy.

Then there is my mother. She is all that I have. We don't have any other family since my father passed. I am an only child, and so was my mother. Her parents died when she was young, and she grew up in foster care.

According to my mother, my father's family didn't like her. When he chose her over his family they stopped talking to him, so I have never met any of them. I don't even know how to contact them. My mother is sketchy on the details about my father's family and becomes upset when I ask about them, so

I don't ask anymore. She and I have been emotionally distant since my father died. I don't know what happened. We seem to be on different paths, but I would never leave her alone. After all, it's only the two of us.

Jasper and my mother don't like each other, but for my benefit they are cordial to each other. My mother thinks I can do better and Jasper thinks my mother is evil. Jasper never goes into detail about why he thinks my mother is evil. All he ever says is that it's the vibe he gets from her.

Neecy reminds herself, I need to get some sleep. I have a busy day tomorrow. If I oversleep I'll be late meeting Monica and she always gives me a hard time when I'm late meeting her.

The next day, Ugh, I need to hurry. This traffic is hideous today...it's going to make me late for lunch with Monica. There must have been an accident for it to be so backed up. Let me give her a call to let her know I'm on my way.

Chapter 2

Life Without Friendship Is Like Life Without Breathing

This child will be late for her own funeral. Neecy is never on time. I don't see how she manages to take care of patients, but they keep coming back, so I guess she is doing something right. Neecy is my ride or die. We met in our junior year of high school, and we have been friends ever since. I remember when we first met–I had just lost my father in a car accident and was struggling, flunking out of school, just having a hard time dealing with his death. My father and I were so close. He would take me out on dates to make sure I knew how a man was supposed to treat me. My father was our world to my mother and me. When he died, it almost killed both of us. It's a miracle that either of us got back to living life.

Thanks to Neecy I gained a desire to want to keep living. There were so many times I wanted to give up, and she wouldn't let me. Neecy was right there with me every step of the way to help me return to sanity. I guess she could relate because her father had passed a few years earlier. As much as she was there for me, she never really talks about her father or his death. I guess that's her way of dealing with it. We all grieve in different ways.

We were roommates throughout college and medical school. We would still be roommates if she had not met Jasper. Once Jasper entered the picture, everything changed. Neecy decided she needed her own place (or Jasper decided for her) so that they could have their privacy. I haven't decided if I like or dislike him. There is something about Jasper I can't put my finger on it. I'm not sure if it's Jasper I don't trust or Neecy's judgment when it comes to her choice of men.

Neecy is super smart when it comes to school. She graduated at the top of our class in both high school and college. But when it comes to choosing men, all her smarts and common sense go out the window. It's as if she puts blinders on to their issues, or whether she's even compatible with them, especially if they make her feel special when they first meet. And please don't let the man tell her he loves her–they're in without any further screening or taking time to get to know them. She dives in, opens her heart, and sometimes her purse, without any requirement for them to prove they deserve a chance. Neecy has been burned several times financially because a man told her he loved her.

The worst was when she co-signed for and got stuck with a car payment on a car she never drove. I love her the same, she has a heart of gold, and if you are her friend, her loyalty to you can't be shaken.

"Well, it's about time you showed up."

"Girl please, I'm only 10 minutes late. Have you ordered?"

"No, I was waiting for you. Waiter, we are ready to order." The waiter smiles because they both started to speak at the same time ordering the same dish. Neecy looks at Monic and says, "you know me better than anyone."

"It's been a week since we talked, have you had any more dreams other than the one last night?"

"Yes, I have had a few, but they haven't been as vivid as the one I had when I called you last night. Sometimes they can seem so real. There have been times when it seems like I can physically feel someone's hands around my neck. "

"Mmmm, and where is Jasper when you are having these dreams, especially the vivid ones?"

"Oh Monica, don't be ridiculous. Jasper is not choking me when I'm sleeping. "

"Okay Neecy, I'm just saying…."

"Can we change the subject please? I don't want to think about my dreams or Jasper right now. I want to enjoy my lunch with my bestie."

"Okay, but promise me you will be careful where Jasper is concerned and that you will get to know him before you let him move in, give him money, etc."

"Monica, stop worrying, I got this. Jasper is a good person, and he loves me."

"That's what you said about Frank before you ended up paying for his car after he disappeared."

"Okay, okay, I hear you. Can we change the subject now? I want to hear all about the new love of your life."

"Well, the new love is an old love or should I say now a past love."

"What! Are you serious? You guys were together for six months. I thought he was going to be a keeper. What happened?"

"Mark just wasn't the one. We started off strong, but he doesn't have any drive or ambition. I just couldn't see myself with him long term."

"Another one bites the dust," Neecy says laughing. At least he lasted longer than the others."

"Well, you know how I feel about wasting time. Some people are only meant to be in our lives for a season and others for a lifetime. Those that are only meant to be here for a season are here to fulfill a purpose in our lives. They show up to teach us something, or to assist us with something, or vice versa. It's our responsibility to recognize those that are only intended to be in our lives for a season and let go when the season is over. "

Neecy interrupts, "I know, I know…when that season is over, but we don't let go, we prolong the

11

pain. We may even miss out on someone that is meant to be in our lives for a lifetime because the person that was only intended to be here for a season is taking up the space of someone that was intended to be in our lives for a lifetime."

"Yasss, you got it. I wish you would practice it more Neecy. I'm really worried about you. The dreams you're having and how Jasper always conveniently sleeps through all of it..."

Neecy interrupts Monica, "I told you, I fully trust Jasper. I don't know...there is something about him that makes me feel safe, like he has been sent to protect me."

"What do you mean to protect you?"

"I don't mean he is there to protect me from danger. He feels safe, as if he is my protector. I feel safe with him."

"I give up Neecy, you won't hear me. I hope he does prove me wrong and he turns out to be the wonderful guy you think he is."

"Hey, when are you going to come to a yoga class with me?"

"Monica, why do we have to keep having this conversation? I don't like yoga. The whole breathing fixation doesn't work for me."

"I'm shocked that you don't think more of breathing techniques and the benefits to your health especially being a doctor."

"It's *because* I'm a doctor. I don't need anyone to teach me how to breathe, we do it naturally."

"Dr. Shanice "Neecy" Stromm, you're hopeless."

"Why thank you Dr. Armstrong."

Monica sighs, "Breathing techniques can reduce stress, anxiety, improve your sleep, and there is scientific proof of other health benefits. Just the other day I was reading an article about the different types of breathing."

"So, are you getting ready to give me a lesson on breathing?"

"Neecy I'm just trying to convince you to try one class with me. I think it will be great for us to do something together, like old times. We hardly get to see each other anymore."

"Oh, would you look at the time, I need to get back to the hospital. I have patients waiting for me. I want to finish my shift on time because Jasper is taking me to dinner."

"Mmm, change the subject for now, but you know what I say about living life on life's terms. You are going to wish you had gone to yoga with me."

"I will go to a class with you...I just have to figure out my schedule. Just know I'm not going because I think I need to learn how to breathe–I've been doing that for 29 years just fine. I do, however, like the idea of being able to spend some time with my bestie."

"You weren't saying that when you called me in the middle of the night, Monica laughs."

Neecy sighs, "I do have to get going, I'm going to stop and check on my mother on my way to the hospital. I'll give you a call tomorrow."

"Ok, I'll have the yoga class schedule."

"Yeah, yeah... "

"Tell your mother I said hello."

Chapter 3

Breathe

"Hi Mama, how are you today?" Neecy leans over to kiss her mother Alice on the cheek.

"Hi Neecy. Neecy you know I don't like it when you wear your hair like that, and for heaven sakes at least put on some lip gloss and eyeliner! What your patients must think."

"Oh Mama, I don't have time for that. Besides, when someone comes into the emergency room for medical treatment, they could care less if I have on eyeliner."

"Child, you are hopeless." "Mama, you are the only woman I know that can wake up looking put together. I don't see how you do it. So, how are you? We haven't talked in a couple of days."

"I'm the same as I was the last time you stopped by to visit. You have just gone on with your life and forgot about me."

"How can you say I've forgotten about you when I call and stop by all the time? If it were up to you, you would have me move back in and never leave the house."

"Would that be asking too much? I want you to move back in with me."

"Mother, we have had this conversation many times, I'm not moving back in. I have my own place, and I'm happy. I like being on my own."

"First it was Monica putting ideas in your head that you should leave me and go to college. Now it's that Jackie."

"It's Jasper Mama."

"Close enough. Now he has filled your head with things and convinced you to get your own place. I bet he gets to visit and probably stay over anytime he likes."

"Mama, you can visit anytime you like…I mean, anytime I'm home."

"That's another thing, all those hours you work, you don't even have time for a conversation with me.

"Mama, I'm here now. What do you want to talk about?"

"Nothing, never mind."

"OK Mama, have it your way. But I do want to talk to you about something."

"What is it?"

"I've been having the dreams again. I —"

"Stop! Stop right there. I don't want to hear about any more of your crazy dreams. Nobody is choking you Neecy, nobody is trying to kill you. You have been having these dreams since you were a child and nothing ever comes of them. You're still here right?"

"Yes Mother, but —"

"But nothing, it's all in your head Neecy. Whenever you are overwhelmed, you start talking about those dreams. When you were a child, whenever you watched a murder/mystery movie you would have those dreams. Stop watching those type of movies and stop letting everything and everybody overwhelm you, and you won't have the dreams!"

"Mama, the dreams must be coming from somewhere. There must be a basis for them. You know Freud said that dreams are the window to our subconscious."

"OMG, not Freud…have you been talking to Monica again? That girl has taken a few psychology courses and now she thinks *she* is Sigmund Freud?" Alice says sarcastically as she waves her hands.

When Alice waves her hands, its Neecy's signal that she is done talking about the subject. However, this time Neecy presses. "Mama, the dreams are becoming more vivid, more real. Sometimes I can feel someone's hands around my neck. I wake up crying and gasping for air."

"Neecy, that's ridiculous to think someone is trying to harm you."

"I know it is, but it keeps happening. There must be something to it, a reasonable explanation."

"Something like what?" Alice asks as she raises an eyebrow.

Neecy knows that when Alice raises one eyebrow (something she has never been able to do, no matter how hard she's tried), she's interested in what Neecy is saying. "Mother, I want to go see someone."

"You want to see someone like who?"

"You know, a therapist."

"A head shrink? You want to go and see a head shrink about a silly dream? Are you kidding me right now? And what do you think a head shrink is going to tell you that I haven't already told you? No child of mine is going to lay on somebody's couch and tell our family business because she had a bad dream. Neecy I forbid it. You will not embarrass me by seeing a head shrink."

"How is my seeing a therapist embarrassing you?" I'm just trying to get to the bottom of these dreams." Neecy starts to back down from the conversation when she sees Alice's face go from interested to upset. Neecy and her father know the wrath of Alice all too well when she gets upset. She goes from 0 to 60 in a matter of seconds. It's like a light switch is flicked on. Alice can be the nicest person you ever want to know, but you don't want to get on her bad side. She has a mean streak that can't be compared to anything Neecy has ever seen before.

When Alice gets mad, Neecy has to remind herself that she is the same person. Neecy has always had a hard time understanding her mother. Outside the home, people love her. She can be so charismatic. People have described her personality as dynamic, sweet, but shy. Neecy always believed that Alice's shyness is why she doesn't have any friends. Alice keeps to herself, never has people over, and she never goes anywhere for entertainment purposes. The funny thing is, she is always dressed like a fashion model. From head to toe, she is always well put together. But when she gets mad, you better not be the one in her path because when she lashes out, you won't even see it coming…and she must win.

Neecy remembers when she was in 8th grade and she was having trouble with math. Alice went to meet with her teacher to figure out how to improve her grade. The teacher made the mistake of telling Alice she could be contributing to Neecy failing math and Alice went ballistic. Alice told the teacher she was incompetent, that she didn't know her head from a hole in the wall and proceeded to belittle her. The school called the police and had a restraining order issued against Alice. She was forbidden to come on school grounds. Neecy remembers being so embarrassed the remainder of the school year. Alice could not attend any of her 8th grade school events.

"OK, Mother, I hear you. I won't see anyone. I'm good. I'll try to reduce my stress level and make sure I'm not watching any movies I shouldn't watch."

"Now that's my girl. Would you like some lunch?"

"No thanks, I just came from lunch with Monica, and I have to get back to the hospital."

"Oh, so the only reason you came over here was to try and convince me you need a head shrink?"

"No Mama, not at all. I stopped by to see you, and it just came up."

"Sure, it just came up. I bet Monica had something to do with it—she put you up to this didn't she? Monica has never been good enough for your friendship. You remember, I am the only real friend you have."

"Mother, it's not Monica. No, she didn't put me up to this. And you are my mother."

"Can't I be your mother and your best friend?"

"Yes, Mother, you are my best friend. I have to go… I'm going to be late getting back." Neecy gives her mother a quick kiss on the cheek and rushes out the door. "Whew! I had to get out of there before she got to 60, I don't feel like dealing with that today."

Neecy is such a beautiful woman. Alice thinks to herself. She has a natural beauty–her skin is perfectly smooth. She was one of those lucky teenagers that never had to deal with acne. She has always been health conscious. I guess that's why I was not surprised when she told me she had decided to go to medical school. As beautiful as that girl is, she drives me crazy. I sometimes wonder how she has made it in this world, especially when she was away at college.

Alice continues to think to herself, at least I was able to convince her to move back home once she graduated and take a job close to me. She wears her heart on her sleeve, lets that hospital overwork her and spends most of her time there. Well, at least she did until that Jasper came along. Unfortunately, she believes there is good in everyone and refuses to see the bad. Even as a child it was difficult to get her not to think everyone was good. Just like her father, humph. That's why when either of them got out of line and thought they were going to run this household, I had to show them. "I'm Queen B and for as long as I live I will be Queen B!" Alice shouts at the door.

Who does she think she is, she owes me her life. Alice thinks out loud. If it weren't for me, she wouldn't be alive right now. She is so much like her father–he was always trusting everyone. That's why I had to control what he did until the day he died.

Otherwise, who knows where we would have ended up. I've always told her, win at all cost. You have no friends when it comes to winning.

I know I give her a hard time about Monica, but, she's harmless. Otherwise, I would have never allowed them to remain friends. But I still have to keep her off her game by making her think I don't care for Monica. Now that Jasper character, he's another story. I don't like him. I don't trust him, and I can't let him get any closer to Neecy. He slipped in on me. Everything would be so much easier if Neecy would just break up with him. The moment I met him I knew what he was, what he is capable of doing. I can't let him infiltrate our lives any further because if he does, it can only go one way for Neecy and me–bad.

It's time to put 'Operation Break-up' into play. In this life, it's about the survival of the fittest, and I am a survivor. Jasper is bad news for us, I can feel it. I know who you are Jasper, I see you. Yeah Jasper, you haven't met the real me yet, but you will, and soon. You can cause a lot of damage to our lives, and I won't allow it. I've survived many, so one more won't make a difference. And trust…. you *will* go away Jasper, one way or another.

Alice smiles as she takes another sip of her drink. As she continues to thinks to herself, she hasn't had to revert to desperate means in a long time and had forgotten how much she enjoyed that life. Getting Jasper out of their lives calls for desperate measures, and she is just the one to deliver them. "Yassss Jasper, Alice says out loud, I'm coming for you, but you won't see me coming. You won't even know what hit you until it's too late."

Chapter 4

Keep Breathing

"Where is she? I've been calling her all day–not even a text that she will call me back. Wait until I see her...I think she is defiant on purpose. I have told her over and over, I need to know where she is, what she's doing, especially when she is not at work. See, this is exactly why I was telling myself not to go there...but it's too late now. I wasn't supposed to fall in love with Neecy, but I did. It just happened, and now I can't get enough of her. Now I get what Rose Royce was talking about in their song "I'm In Love":

> *Just one look, that's all it took*
> *I was hooked, from the very start*
> *And the feeling's wonderful, marvelous, heavenly,*
> *You're ecstasy*
>
> *My heart feels light like a bird in flight I won't need*
> *any air, yeah, yeah.......*
> *Hey, I'm in love*

Neecy is ecstasy for me. I've never felt this way about a woman, any women. I didn't think it was even possible for me to feel this way about a woman.

I used to go to the hospital and pretend I was visiting someone so that I could watch her. The first time I saw Neecy, I knew we were meant to be together. I wasn't sure she would give me the time of day, but I was determined to make her mine. I love her more than life itself, but I can't trust her. You know how women are–manipulative, cunning and most are whores, just looking for a man to take care of them. They are willing to do anything necessary to get a man, even if it means spending most of their time on their backs. But Neecy was different...that's what attracted me to her.

I used to watch her in the hospital cafeteria, the way she chewed her food, the kind of food she liked, her favorite meal and how she liked her coffee. When I would go up to the hospital to watch her, I watched the men panting behind her, and she would pretend she didn't notice so that she could draw them in. I have to remind myself often that I can't trust her. Her sweet ways, her friendliness and her big heart are all a part of her ploy, her manipulation to keep men panting at her feet.

Women in general can't be trusted. All my life I watched the women in my family manipulate men to satisfy their needs. I had to take care of my two younger brothers because my mother was always too busy "entertaining" men. My mother didn't have a real job. Her job was to entertain men. She couldn't be bothered with making sure she took care of us.

All I grew up around were women that never worked. They had male friends that provided for them. I had more "uncles" than any child should ever have. I couldn't keep up with who my uncle of the day was, there were so many. Not to mention not all uncles are good uncles. In fact, some uncles provided for my mother so that they could have access to her boys.

Some of my uncles used to treat my mother like trash. I couldn't stand to watch them belittle her, and some would even beat her. One time I tried to stop "Uncle Sam" from beating my mother. It was late one night, I had just turned 13, and I had just gotten my younger brothers in bed when the violence erupted. I heard Uncle Sam yelling "get rid of it! Then my mother screamed, and I ran in the room just in time to see my Uncle Sam punching my mother in the stomach. I grabbed my baseball bat and told him if he hit her again I was going to beat him with it. He laughed, pushed me down and asked me what I was going to do. I swung my bat but missed, and he pushed me down again.

To my surprise, my mother grabbed her belt and threatened to beat me with it if I didn't stay out of her business. She chastised me for swinging my bat at Uncle Sam. After she beat me with her belt, she made me go to bed. I heard her begging Uncle Sam not to leave. I never tried to protect my mother again, despite all the "Uncle Sam's that followed.

Shortly after my 18th birthday, I moved out but would go by daily to check on my brothers. One night I got a frantic phone call from my brother asking me to come over right away. When I got there, the police and ambulance were already there. The paramedics were there trying to revive my mother. Blood was everywhere, and my mother laid lifeless on the living room floor with my brothers watching in horror as the paramedics tried to revive her.

The story goes, my mother had just sent my brothers to bed when they heard her screaming. At first, they just tried to go to sleep because it wasn't out of the norm to hear our mother screaming. But then they heard her scream in a way they had never heard before. They ran into the room in time to see our latest uncle pull the knife out of her chest and stab her again. They ran next door to the neighbor who called the police. The police arrested the man for murder. He killed my mother for taking $20 out of his pocket after he fell asleep. You see why women can't be trusted? My mother lost her life for stealing $20 from a man who was supposed to care about her. There is one thing that I did learn from all my "uncles"–the man should always be in control of the relationship.

"Hi sweetie, how are you?" Neecy's voice breaks through Jasper's thoughts as she walks through the door.

"Don't sweetie me." Jasper snaps. "I've been calling and texting you all day."

"Well hello to you too Jasper. I've been busy all day. The emergency room has been buzzing. I don't know if it's a full moon or what, but it's been non-stop."

"You couldn't take two minutes and send me a text?"

"Jasper, you are going overboard, I was busy."

"The emergency room couldn't have been that busy because I stopped by during your lunch break. Karen told me you had gone out for lunch."

"Karen and her big mouth." Neecy thinks to herself. "Jasper, relax. I just met Monica for lunch. It's been a while since I've seen her and we wanted to catch up. Is that what this is about, you think I was out with someone else?"

"No, I know better than that. I just can't figure out why you can't respond when I text or call but you can make time for Monica."

"Are you trying to piss me off Jasper? Monica is my best friend, and we hadn't seen each other in a while."

"You told me you guys just went to lunch last week."

"We did. Going a week without hanging out with her seems like a while, especially since she is my best friend. We have been inseparable since high school. Are you jealous of Monica?"

Jasper makes and face. "Don't give her so much credit. I don't like Monica...she's always calling, trying to get you to go somewhere or hang out, and it takes time from us."

"Don't be ridiculous, seeing Monica for a couple of hours once a week is not taking time from us."

"I guess I'm the reason you don't see your mother as much too?

"Now that you mention it, I did stop by my mother's today. She was in one of her moods, so I didn't stay long."

"You mean one of her evil spells?"

"Jasper, that's not nice, and don't talk about my mother like that."

"Neecy, I know that's your mother, but I'm telling you, there is something about her I haven't figured out yet that makes me uncomfortable. Anyway, my point is you can make time for them, but you can't take 2 minutes to text me back."

Neecy is exasperated. "Jasper, I just saw you this morning. We see each other almost every day. It's only been a few hours."

"Damn it Neecy, stop arguing with me and do what I tell you! Especially when it has to do with your mother...I don't trust her."

"Why don't you trust my mother? Where is that coming from? My mother raised me, and she has gotten me this far without incident, so don't tell me I can't go and see her. In fact, you don't tell me *who* I can see or talk to. You are my boyfriend, not my father."

"Go all day again without responding to my call or text."

"Now wait a minute Jasper, you are taking things way too far, and don't yell at me again. I'm not your child, I'm your girlfriend…soon to be ex-girlfriend if you don't lighten up. I'm not your mother.

"What did you say? Say it again!" yells Jasper, grabbing Neecy's arm.

"Jasper let me go!" screams Neecy trying to shake her arm loose.

"Say it again!" Jasper yells at her.

"I'm sorry, I took that too far." Neecy says as Jasper lets go of her arm. "I shouldn't have said anything about your mother…I know that's a sensitive issue. It was wrong of me to bring that up and use it against you. It won't happen again. But let me be clear, if you ever grab my arm again, especially when we are arguing, we are done. I don't care what has been done or said."

"You're right, I'm sorry too. I get so crazy when I don't hear from you. I start to think the worst, and I don't think I could stand it if I ever lost you."

"I'm not going anywhere Jasper. I don't know how else to assure you of that. I need you to stop being so dramatic and overbearing...you're smothering me."

"Smothering you? That's what you think, I'm smothering you? Don't answer my calls again, and I'll show you smothering. Do you hear me Neecy?"

"I can't do this right now. Forget dinner...I need some space." Neecy grabs her keys and runs out the door. Jasper follows yelling for her to come back. As she watches the house grow smaller in her rear-view mirror, Neecy gets lost in her thoughts.

As she pulls in front of her cabin, she says out loud, "I didn't think I would ever get here. I can't remember if I have clean linen...doesn't matter...I'm exhausted. After all these years, this door still sticks, every time I come up here I tell myself I need to get it fixed. A little elbow, mph, whew, I didn't think I was going to get it opened." Neecy walks into the room looking around, just the way I left it. I'll get water in the morning.

Chapter 5

Breath is the Secret of Life

Neecy falls asleep on the couch and wakes with the sun shining brightly through the window. She stretches to help wake up and then goes outside and takes in deep breaths.

I always loved coming up here to the mountains, the air is so fresh, and this time of year is so beautiful. Trees are blooming, flowers and wildlife all about. I could retire up here or at least hide out for a long time. I miss coming up here with my father. This was our spot. We would come up here when my mother was on a rampage or in one of her moods. This is my place of serenity. When I come here, all my problems seem so small. I can think and be free of any worries or concerns. After my father died, I purchased this place to always remind me of him, our special place.

Our one rule was that we could only talk about negative things on the way here and on the way home, but when we were here, this was a place of serenity. We could only talk and think about good things, positive thoughts that made us happy. I miss him so much. "God why did you take him from me? He was my best friend." I could talk to my father about anything. I could tell him about the worst of me, and he was never judgmental, never stopped loving me.

Those times when we were getting away from my mother, we would come up here and stay for days. He would let me run, play and be free. I could even use the bathroom in the woods. Then at night, we would build a fire in the fireplace and roast marshmallows. Sometimes we would pretend we were in an old western movie cooking out on the prairie. We would sing old western songs like "Home on the Range. Neecy starts singing to herself

"Oh, give me a home where the buffalo roam,
Where the deer and the antelope play,
Where seldom is heard a discouraging word,
And the skies are not cloudy all day…"

Neecy begins to cry. Although her dad has been gone for years, she still talks to him as if he were there, "Why did you leave me?" "Didn't you know I still needed you…?" But then she starts to hear her mother tell her to stop crying. Her mother would say that as long as her daddy has been dead, she should be over it…she should be done crying about him being gone. Neecy thinks to herself, I don't know if you can put a timeline on grief. Grief is personal. Each person deals with it differently and for some it's more present at certain times depending on who you are grieving and under what circumstances.

There are times I don't think about my father, but those times that I do—the times I really miss him— are usually during those special times in my life. Like when I graduated from high school and college, when I got my white coat. Those are the times that I miss him most, when I long for him to be there, to share in those moments with me. I know my mother and I don't agree, but I think it's okay to miss my father during those special times. His love was unconditional.

I remember when I first got the news that my father had died. At first, I couldn't believe it. I refused to believe he was gone. I just went numb. I couldn't feel anything. Sometimes I still feel that way, hoping that there has been some mistake…hoping he will walk through the door one day. And when he doesn't, I become angry. Angry at him for leaving me, angry at God for taking him.

There are days I start to miss my father, and I can barely get out of bed. There are those days I just want to curl up and join him, but then I tell myself he's not coming back and life must go on. So I force myself out of bed. I force myself to continue with the day. I haven't prayed since the day of my father's funeral. Pray for what? God didn't answer my prayer back then—He didn't bring my father back. God and I have had nothing to talk about since that day." Neecy is now yelling at the sky, "What kind of God takes from you the only person that has ever truly loved you? What God allows you to carry this type of pain?"

"Neecy are you ok?" Neecy jumps up from the stump she was sitting on, startled, with tears streaming down her face.

"Jasper, what are you doing here? How did you find me?"

"I followed you last night and slept in the car at the bottom of the hill."

"Now you're stalking me?" "No Neecy, it's nothing like that, I'm not stalking you. You left so abruptly and I didn't know where you were going or if you were okay, so I followed you here. I saw you pull up to the cabin and I parked at the bottom of the hill and slept in the car."

Neecy snaps at Jasper, you had no right to come here. If I wanted you here, I would have invited you.

"What is this place Neecy?" Jasper asks looking around the property.

"It's none of your business......now leave!"

"Neecy I'm not leaving you up here by yourself."

"Jasper, I want you to leave right now. I told you I needed some space. Leave me alone...leave me alone for good."

"What does that mean?"

"It means exactly what you think it means—we are done Jasper. I'm tired of you smothering me. I can't move without you blowing up my phone, texting and calling all day. If I don't pick up the phone, you're coming by my job, my house. I never get a break from you."

"And now this! You followed me here? Leave this place and leave me alone. I will call you when I get back to the city so that you can come and get your things."

"Neecy, you don't mean that. You don't want to break up with me, you don't know what you're saying."

"I know exactly what I'm saying. Leave!"

"Fine Neecy, I'll leave, but this isn't over. We are going to talk when you get back."

"There's nothing to talk about Jasper. Leave!

I can't believe he followed me up here. He's ruined my serenity. I might as well head back. Neecy's thoughts are interrupted by the smell of smoke, something burning. Neecy looks around and sees a flame coming from behind the cabin.

"Oh my God, is the cabin on fire?" As she turns to run to the cabin, she runs into someone and is startled. "Jasper what are you still doing here?"

"Neecy I can't just leave it like this, I need you to listen to me."

"Jasper, I don't have time for this, something is burning. The cabin is on fire!"

"Neecy, you are going to listen to me!" he says grabbing her.

"Jasper let me go!

"No, I'm not letting you go until you listen to me."

"Let me go now! I mean it let me go!" Neecy breaks loose from Jasper's grip and runs towards the cabin. Jasper follows her and grabs her just as she reaches the porch.

"Jasper let me go!"

"Neecy, you are going to listen to me!"

"No, I'm not! Let…me…go! I don't want you here. In fact, I don't want *you*! Let me go. My cabin is on fire! Let me go!"

Chapter 6

You Are Where You Need To Be, Just Take A Deep Breath
~ Lana Parrilla ~

"This is the third time I've called you today Neecy, where are you? This is the second day in a row that I've called and left messages, and you haven't called me back. I'm standing here with Karen. She also left you a message this morning to see if you can come in earlier than your scheduled shift today and you haven't returned her call. Yesterday was your day off, but you're not calling back, and this is not like you. I'm getting worried. Please call me by noon, or I'm going to file a missing person's report.'

"Jasper, this is Monica, the hospital and I have been trying to reach Neecy since yesterday. This is the second message I have left you. If you have seen Neecy or know why she is not answering her phone, please give me a call. I'm getting worried about her."

"Karen, I'm not sure what's going on. If I hear from her, I will call you and vice versa. If she calls in, please call me."

"One second Dr. Armstrong, I have ambulance duty. The paramedics are calling in. While I take this call, can you write down your number so I won't have to look it up."

"Here you go Karen, I'm headed home. You can reach me at this number if you hear from her." Monica says as she hands Karen the slip of paper.

"Thanks Dr. Armstrong. I will."

Karen listens to ambulance message coming through, "Nurse, alert the emergency room doctor to be on standby, we have an ambulance coming in. ETA 2 mins. They have a female approximately 30 years of age rescued from a fire. She has smoke inhalation, a stab wound, and has lost a lot of blood." Karen takes charge giving orders and informing the emergency room staff of the arrival of the ambulance. "The ambulance is here. Everyone, stand by. Dave, what do you guys have for us today?"

"Nurse Karen, I didn't want to say this over the radio, but I think you know the patient."

"What? I know the patient...who is it?"

Dave looks over his shoulder, "We are bringing her in now."

"Oh My God! Nurse, call Mr. Anderson!"

"Mr. Anderson, the Hospital Administrator?"

"What other Mr. Anderson would I tell you to call? Tell him we are admitting one of our own into the emergency room...it's Dr. Stromm! Dave do you know what happened?"

"No, not exactly. We responded to a call for a house fire, and as we were pulling up, the fireman was carrying her out. She has a stab wound and her vitals are weak. It was touch and go for a minute. I didn't think she was going to make it. Her face is swollen and bruised as if she was in a fight. I was pretty sure it was Dr. Stromm, but I didn't want to say over the radio just in case it wasn't her. The other person in the house was burned beyond recognition."

"Oh my goodness! Thanks Dave."

"Hey Nurse Karen, will you keep us posted?" asks Dave. "Dr. Stromm is one of our favorites. All the paramedics know we were bringing her in…we would like to know when she pulls through."

"Yes, of course, I'll let you know. I have to go. We have a Doctor to save." Dave nods and walk over to the nurse's station to hang around.

"Nurse Karen, get her in OR #5, stat, and get her blood type down here stat, she has lost a lot of blood. We are going to have to move fast if she is going to have a fighting chance. Yes Dr. Turner, I'm on it. Karen yells over her shoulder, "Nurse Nancy, can you call her next of kin and Dr. Armstrong? Dr. Armstrong just left the nurse's station…see if you can catch her in the parking lot.

Nancy takes off running toward the parking lot, "Dr. Armstrong! Dr. Armstrong! Wait!" Nancy yells running toward Monica.

"My goodness, Nancy, I've never seen you move so fast. Take a minute to catch your breath."

"No time." Nancy says in between breaths, "it's Dr. Stromm."

"What about her? Did she finally show up?"

"Dr. Armstrong, come with me, it's Dr. Stromm. The paramedics brought her into the emergency room."

"What? The emergency room!"

They both take off running back into the hospital as fast as their legs will carry them. When Monica gets to the nurse's station, Karen is coming around the corner. "Karen, what's going on?"

"Dr. Stromm has been admitted. The ambulance brought her into the emergency room after you walked away? She was rescued from a house fire, there is smoke inhalation, but that's not the worst.

"The worst?"

"She has a stab wound and has lost a lot of blood."

"What? I need to see her!".

"You can't right now. She is in the OR. Dr. Turner is the surgeon. You know Dr. Turner is one of our best, and he happened to be on duty, so she is in good hands. All we can do is wait."

Monica's head is spinning. "This can't be real... Nancy tells Monica that Dave was the paramedic on the scene and who brought her in. "Dave, what happened?" Monica asks as she fights back the tears.

"Doctor we responded to a two-alarm house fire, when we got there, they were carrying Dr. Stromm out. The other person in the house was already deceased, burned beyond recognition. There was nothing we could do."

"Do you remember the address?" asks Monica.

"Yes, the house was on Staples St."

"This is not happening...this can't be happening."

"What Dr. Armstrong, what is it?"

"That's the street that Dr. Stromms' mother lives on."

Monica collapses in the paramedic's arms with tears streaming down her face. The emergency room staff is temporarily paralyzed where they are standing. Nobody is speaking. No one knows what to say. All you can hear is the sound of sniffling as tissues are being passed around. After a few seconds go by, what seems likes hours, Nurse Karen finally announces to the hospital staff in the room, "we still have other patients." Dr. Armstrong if you want to wait in the Doctors' lounge, I will let you know as soon as I hear something." Dave speaks up and says he can sit with Dr. Armstrong until he gets another emergency call.

Dr. Armstrong thanks Dave in between tears. She tries again to call Jasper, but it goes straight to voicemail. Monica keeps saying, "I have to pray for her, I have to pray. Nurse Nancy, I'll be in the chapel. As Monica enters the chapel, she rushes to the altar. Dave sits in the back pew and bows his head. Monica begins to pray out loud.

"My most heavenly and precious father, I come to you with a bowed head and humble heart. Lord, you know the beginning and the end. Please God, don't let this be the end for Neecy. Don't take her away from us, from me, I don't think my heart can handle it. Father, we ask for your healing hands in the operating room. I ask that you touch, rule and abide in Neecy's circumstances, guide the surgeon's hands, have your way in the operating room. Keep her and keep breathing life into her. I pray for the complete and total healing of Neecy, mind, body, and soul. I thank you, and I give you the praise that it's already done. In Jesus name…" Dave gives a quiet amen from the back pew.

Chapter 7

Running on Air

Meanwhile, in the operating room, Dr. Turner is calling out orders. "Let's get her on the table. Nurse, do you have the x-rays? I need to see how deep the wound is and if any vital organs were hit." Dr. Turner takes a deep breath after reviewing the x-rays and announces to the room a lung has been punctured. "I can't tell from the x-ray how much damage has been done. Be on standby in case the lung collapses. Nurse, scalpel!"

Once in, Dr. Turner takes another deep breath and announces, no serious damage done, the blade just nicked the lung. He whispers, "Your God was with you today Dr. Neecy Stromm."

Dr. Turner continues to give orders, "Let's get the blood flowing, get this wound cleaned up and treat her for the smoke inhalation." Dr. Turner leans over and whispers in Neecy's ear, "You're not out of the woods yet Dr. Stromm, but I know you are determined and you're a fighter. Fight to come back to us." He looks up at the operating room staff, "Close her up. I'm going to talk to the family.

"Nurse Karen, where's the family?" Karen takes a deep sigh to hold back the tears. As a tear falls, she tells Dr. Turner that the detectives have arrived and are waiting to talk to him. She explains that Dr. Stromm was rescued from her mother's burning house. Her mother wasn't so lucky and what is believed to be her mother's body was burned beyond recognition. She was Dr. Stromm's next of kin. Dr. Armstrong is also listed as an emergency contact. Then Karen remembers Monica is in the chapel and tells Dr. Turner she is waiting to hear the prognosis. Okay, let me talk to Monica first and then the detectives.

Monica is still praying and doesn't see Dr. Turner enter the chapel, but Dave rushes to meet him. Dr. Turner touches Monica's shoulder. She looks up at him with fresh and dried tears streaming down her face. Mike, how is she? Please tell me she is going to be okay. Neecy is not out of the woods yet, but she did tolerate the surgery well. She is a fighter. I think she is going to pull through."

"Thank God! When can I see her?"

"I'm having her moved to ICU right now. I want to take extra precautions to make sure she pulls through."

Monica nods her head as the tears fall. Dave shakes the doctor's hand and announces to no one in particular that he has to go but will let the other paramedics know she pulled through. Monica rushes to ICU to wait for them to bring Neecy to her room. While waiting, she calls Jasper again, but this time Monica tells him since he's not answering his phone he must have had something to do with hurting Neecy. Monica threatens to hunt him down and assures him she won't stop looking for him until she finds him. Justice will be served.

The word spreads throughout the hospital that Dr. Stromm pulled through the surgery. As the news spread you begin to hear cheers, claps and "thank you Gods" throughout the corridors. Everyone loves Neecy and everyone had taken pause to say a prayer, send positive vibes and listen for the news. Monica is sitting with Neecy when the detective walks in. Hello, I'm Detective Sherman. Ma'am I know the victim hasn't woken up yet, but I understand that you are her best friend? Monica nods. "Would you be willing to answer some questions?"

Monica nods again, "Yes, of course."

"Ma'am, do you know of anyone that would want to hurt the victim." the detective asks.

"The victim's name is Dr. Shanice Stromm, she goes by Neecy."

"Yes, of course. I didn't mean any disrespect." "Do you have any idea of who would want to hurt Dr. Stromm?"

As Monica answers yes, she takes off running past the detective. "You didn't have to hurt her! What did you do! Why did you hurt her!" As Monica is hitting Jasper, the staff and the detective try to restrain her. Monica keeps yelling, "Why would you do this to her!"

While Jasper is trying to move out of the way of Monica's fist, he yells he hasn't hurt anyone. "He yells at Monica that she is crazy…. you're crazy!" By now Detective Sherman and hospital security are standing between them.

Detective Sherman tells them if they don't calm down, they can tell their sides of the story at the police station. Monica takes a deep breath and says Jasper had to be the one to hurt Neecy and her mother.

As the emergency room staff celebration of Neecy pulling through the surgery is coming to an end, they look up and are frozen in their tracks by who they see standing at the nurse's station.

"Dr. Stromm? Dr. Stromm is that you?"

"Yes." Neecy says laughing. "Karen what's wrong? You look like you have just seen a ghost. Is my new hairstyle that bad?"

"Dr. Stromm, we have been calling you for two days…you…you didn't respond"

"Yes, I know. I had something personal going on, and I just needed some time. I haven't had a chance to check my messages, but I'm here in time for my shift."

"Dr. Stromm, I think you need to sit down."

"What, why do I need to sit, what's going on? I heard you guys had some excitement this afternoon. One of our own was admitted to the hospital?" "Oh, no." Neecy can feel her heart start racing, is that why you want me to sit down? Is it someone we worked with? Do I know them?"

Karen is still staring at Neecy when she answers, "Yes, well no, I'm not sure if you know the person admitted today."

"Karen what kind of answer is that, what's going on?"

"Dr. Stromm, the person we admitted today was you."

Neecy starts laughing a sigh of relief and confusion. "What do you mean you admitted me? I'm standing right here."

"Dr. Stromm, we admitted a lady that looks just like you."

"There must be some mistake. Karen, as you can see, I'm standing right here."

"Yes, but everyone thought it was you, even the paramedics that brought you in thought it was you."

"Because she had some resemblance, you all just assumed it was me?"

"No Dr. Stromm she looks like you, not a resemblance, she is the same height, same skin color, same hair. We thought it was you. And there is more…."

"More, what do you mean more? What, she had my ID or something?"

"No Dr. Stromm…you know what, let me call Dr. Armstrong, she is upstairs in ICU with the person we thought was you."

"So not even my best friend could tell that the person wasn't me? No don't call her down, I will go up, I want to see this person."

Chapter 8

Air Is Vital If You Want to Breathe

Neecy turns and heads towards the elevators before Karen can respond. As Neecy approaches the nurse's station, they all freeze where they stand. As Neecy approaches one of the nurses, she is barely able to say, "Dr. Stromm."

"Yes, it's me. I'm not sure who you have in ICU, but I'm here to find out. What room is she in?" The nurse tries to talk, but nothing will come out, so she points as Neecy walks toward the room. The woman is lying there unconscious. When Neecy sees her, all she can do is stare.

"Who is this woman." Neecy says to herself? "I know people say that we all have a twin, but this is a bit much?" As Neecy is staring at the woman, she hears a voice behind her call her name. As she turns, Monica runs and hugs her so hard they almost fall. Monica is sobbing and touching Neecy's face, "Is it you, is it really you?"

"Yes, it's me, Monica! Can you let me go, you are squeezing the air out of me."

"I'm so sorry Neecy! I thought it was you over there in that bed." "Well, obviously it's not…but who is *she*?"

"I think we should wait until she wakes before we say any more." Jasper interrupts.

"I agree with him Neecy" says Monica. I just spent the last hour with Jasper and Detective Sherman. I think we should wait until she is awake so that we can verify who she is so that we don't cause any more confusion.

Neecy looks around the room and back and forth at Jasper and Monica. She says, "Normally I would protest and demand to know what you know right now. However, just the fact that the two of you are agreeing and up until a few minutes ago, everyone thought that was me lying in that bed tells me I need to heed to your advice. And who are you?" Neecy says looking at the Detective Sherman."

"I am Detective Sherman."

"Why is a detective here? I read her chart…is it because you're investigating her stabbing?"

"Yes, Dr. Stromm that's part of the reason I'm here."

"What's the other part? Oh…don't tell me…we should wait until she is awake?"

"Yes ma'am, I'm afraid so."

Neecy sighs, "Okay then, we will wait. But the curiosity is killing me."

Monica looks at Neecy and becomes tearful again. "Neecy, I have something to tell you. I think we should go somewhere else. Let's go to your office so that we can talk."

"I'm coming with you." Jasper says in a matter-of-fact voice.

"I don't know that I'm ready to talk to you Jasper."

"Whether you are ready to talk to me or not—" Monica interrupts Jasper, "Neecy, I think you should let him come with us." Neecy looks at Jasper then back at Monica, trying to determine if she is the only one confused. "I want to know what is going on right now! The two of you are agreeing. Monica you're encouraging me to let Jasper come with us. I want to know right here and right now what's going on because there is obviously a secret that everybody knows but me."

"Neecy please." begs Monica, "let's go to your office where it's private. We will tell you what we know. Agreed, Jasper."

"Yes, agreed." Jasper nods.

"Ok, we will go to my office, but I want to know everything the both of you know. Let me stop by the nurse's station because I want them to let me know the minute this woman opens her eyes."

"What woman are they talking about? Are they talking about me? I can hear voices, but I can't see anyone. I can't tell if my eyes are open or if I'm blind. Hello, can you hear me? Hey, over here! I can hear you talking. Who are these people, where am I?" Angela struggles to move, but can't lift her arms, her legs. "Hey, people, I can hear you. "What's going on, what happened? My name is not woman, it's Angela, Angela McMichael. Don't leave, I can hear you talking…"

"Nurse, I've cleared it with the attending physician—I'm going to my office, but I want to know the minute she is awake. Page me if you have to."

"Yes, Dr. Stromm, I will make sure the incoming shift knows."

"Speaking of the shift, I forgot all about mine! I'm supposed to be on call in the emergency room…our talk will have to wait."

"Monica grabs Neecy's hand, Neecy calm down, they already called someone in to cover your shift. Let's go to your office."

Chapter 9

Sometimes, All You Can Do Is Take A Deep Breath

As they close the door to Neecy's office, she says "Okay, what's going on?"

Monica takes a deep breath, "Neecy, I think you should sit down."

"I don't want to sit down. I want someone to tell me what's going on and why everyone is tiptoeing around me. I want to know now!"

Monica looks at Jasper, and Jasper nods for Monica to go ahead. "Neecy we thought the women in ICU was you because she looks like you."

"Well duh, I've figured that much out."

"We didn't question the identity because the paramedics also thought it was you. They responded to a two-alarm house fire. Monica hesitates and then says through tears; the woman upstairs was rescued from a burning house on Staples Street?"

"Staples Street, my mother lives on Staples Street." "Is it someone I know?" Then, all at once it dawns on Neecy, "Oh My God! Has something happened to my mother? Is she here in the hospital?"

"No Neecy, she is not here."

"Then where is she or was the street just a coincidence?".

Monica takes a deep breath, "No, not a coincidence Neecy." The house was your mother's house. The fireman was not able to save your mother…the body was burned beyond recognition."

"What, my mother is dead?" Neecy exclaims. No, I don't believe you. Really, what's going on?"

"Neecy, you have known me practically all our lives. You know I would never joke about anything like this."

"Nooooooo! Nooooo! Nooooo! She can't be!" Neecy falls to her knees and begins to cry uncontrollably. Neither Monica or Jasper can console her. Through her blurry tears, she asked what happened? How did the fire start? Then it dawns on her that the woman in ICU was in the house. "Did that woman do something to my mother? I'm going to wake her right now!"

"Neecy, she is a weak, and the next 24 hours will be critical, you can't talk to her right now."

"I won't wait! I'll wake her up, and if she did something to my mother, I'm going to put her in a real coma."

Jasper is sitting on the floor with Neecy holding her, "Neecy, we need you to calm down. We don't have the full story, so at this point, the police aren't sure what happened. Your mother may have tried to harm her."

"What!" Neecy jerks away from Jasper, "You would love that wouldn't you? You never liked my mother. Blame the victim."

"No baby, none of this makes me happy, and if you think I take some twisted pleasure in seeing you in this type of pain, you don't know me at all."

"I'm sorry Jasper, I just can't believe she is gone." Neecy is crying again, her entire body shaking. Jasper and Monica have joined her on the floor to console her.

Jasper breaks the silence after a few minutes, "Once she wakes, we will know more about what happened and who she is."

"How can you be so sure?" Neecy asks."

"I'm not sure…I just think she should be able to tell us something "No, Jasper, I know you, you said in a matter-of-fact tone that once she wakes she will be able to tell us more. Do you know who she is?"

Jasper looks away and then at Monica. "Go ahead Jasper, or whatever your name is. You've already given it away, so we might as well tell her what we already know."

Wait, Monica, what do you mean whatever his name is? Your name is Jasper, Jasper Jackson, right? RIGHT?"

"No, not exactly, my real name is Miles Jasper Jackson. My mother loved Miles Davis so she named me after him."

Neecy looks at him in disbelief. "So, you have been lying to me all this time, for months? You have been lying to me about who you are? Why? I want to know why?"

Miles takes a deep breath. "I was hired to find you."

"Find me…I haven't been lost. Who hired you to "find me?"

"I think I was hired by the woman upstairs in ICU. And now seeing her, I'm pretty sure it's her." says Jasper.

"How can you be sure?"

"Because when she hired me, she said she needed me to find her sister."

"I don't have a sister, I'm an only child. I know who my parents were. Neecy pauses, "I said were… this is too much… my mother's gone, my father gone, the love of my life has been lying to me. I don't know who you are, and now you're telling me I may have a sister?"

"I'm pretty sure it's her Neecy."

"How can you be sure Jasper, or Miles, or whatever your name is?"

Miles takes a deep breath, "Neecy, I'm not an engineer, I'm a private detective."

"What! More lies! Oh my God!! I don't know you at all."

"Neecy, you do know me, you know the person I am. I have never let a woman in the way I've let you in, the secrets I've shared with you…the time we have spent together was as real as it gets for me. You may not have known my real name, but you know me the man better than anyone has ever known me."

"Is your little speech supposed to make me feel special? You have been lying to me from day one. Now you want me to believe I know you, that you love me? If I didn't need answers right now, I'd call security."

"Neecy, I think you need to hear him out before you shut him out."

"What, Monica, you're taking his side? What the hell is going on?"

"Neecy, just hear him out and don't make any rash decisions right now, there will be time making decision. Right now, we need to get through this."

"We Monica? We need to get through this? Who is we? What is it you need to get through? Did your mother just die? Did you find out the love of your life has been lying to you the whole time you have been together? Did you have someone tell you they think you have a sister, which by the way, is impossible?"

Monica walks over to Neecy, embraces her and whispers in her ear, "Remember what you told me when my father died?" Neecy looks at Monica and begins to cry uncontrollably. "I'm sorry Monica, I didn't mean any of what I just said, I'm sorry." Neecy says in between tears. Monica hugs Neecy even tighter until she stops crying and asks her if she is okay to allow Miles to go on with his story?" Neecy nods and looks at Miles.

"Neecy, I do love you, heart and soul, you are my—."

"Oh stop, Miles. I can't do this right now. I want you to continue telling me who that woman is upstairs."

Chapter 10

Breath Is Silent Unless You Listen For It

The voice come over the Hospital PA system, "Dr. Stromm, paging Dr. Stromm, please pick up on line 1."

"Hold that thought Miles, let me answer this page. "Yes, this is Dr. Stromm. Thank you nurse, I'm on my way." As Neecy hangs up, she says it was the ICU nurse, the women is awake. As Neecy hurries out the door toward the elevator, she says over her shoulder, "Let's get down to the bottom of this." Monica and Miles quickly follow behind her.

As Neecy, Monica, and Miles enter the room, the attending physician is finishing his exam. Can she talk? She is still weak, and she has lost a lot of blood, but she keeps asking for someone named Miles. Neecy and Monica turn and look at Miles. Miles looks away embarrassed, and then his face changes to a look Neecy has never seen before. She is not sure what Miles is thinking. Miles walks over to the bed, touches the women's hand and says, "I'm here, Miles is here."

The women struggles to open her eyes. When she see's Miles, she smiles. Miles squeezes her hand and the women smiles and closes her eyes. Neecy is glaring at Miles and tells him he better start talking.

"Neecy, she must be scared to death being here and not knowing anyone. I was reassuring her that someone was here, that's all."

"Start talking Miles, or you will be the next one that will need a doctor."

"Okay." Miles continues his story from earlier, "over a year ago, I was contacted by a woman who said she wanted to hire me to find her sister, but I never met her. She said she lived in North Carolina but was pretty sure her sister lived here in Colorado. She gave me some details about the person she wanted me to find, and we set up monthly payments. When I started, I was required to give her monthly updates on my progress. Once I found you, she required that I give her weekly updates. When I notified her that I was sure I had found her sister, which is you, she told me she was coming to Colorado. She didn't want me to tell you who I was or that she was looking for you until she could verify it was you."

"She didn't give me a lot of details, but said she had to make sure it was you before she told you who she was because she wasn't sure how you would respond to the news of her being your sister. She called me two days ago and left a message that she had arrived and told me where she was staying. I was going to meet with her so that she could fill me in on the rest of the story. She also shared with me that she was concerned you had suffered some significant trauma. I was going to tell you about her the night we got into an argument and you left."

"Neecy is screaming at Miles, "Oh, how convenient! You were going to tell me but we got into an argument. And finding me required you to act as if you cared about me, to sleep in my bed, to become the love of my life?"

"Neecy I do care about you. Falling in love with you was not supposed to happen. It wasn't part of the plan"

"And you want me to believe that?"

Monica interrupts, "Let's stay on one subject at a time. Neecy I think you need to hear the rest of what Miles has to say."

"Okay fine...well what did she mean I have suffered some significant trauma? I haven't suffered anything."

Monica interrupts, "I'm not so sure Neecy, I've always suspected you had suffered from some trauma but since I wasn't sure I didn't want to start asking questions and trigger something when I didn't know what I was dealing with."

"Monica gets serious. Why would you think I've suffered from some trauma, and why wouldn't I remember it?"

Monica explains, "That's it Neecy, trauma is subjective, and can impact individuals in different ways. When someone is exposed to a traumatic event, the first days and weeks following can include fear, sadness, guilt, anger, or grief.

However, as they begin to make sense of what has happened to them, these feelings usually begin to subside. Most people will recover quickly, but for some, a traumatic event can lead to mental health issues such as post-traumatic stress disorder (PTSD), depression, anxiety, alcohol and drug use, etc."

"Ok, but I don't have any of that going on so what would make you think I've experienced some traumatic experience?"

Monica takes a deep breath, "For some, the traumatic event can be so severe that they partially, and sometimes completely, block the memory."

"Oh, that's ridiculous Monica." Neecy says laughing. "You have taken too many psychology classes. How can I forget if something has happened to me? After all, I would have been there."

"Neecy this is serious, I need for you to hear me. You have shared with me on numerous occasions you can't remember parts of your life when you were six and your memories prior to age six are foggy at best?"

"Yeah, but my point is I was six. Who remembers details of their life at 6?"

"Most do, maybe not details like you would remember yesterday, but Neecy, you have lost or, should I say, forgotten, almost an entire year. I even tried to talk to your mother about it once, but she got upset, almost ballistic and told me to mind my business or she would make sure we didn't continue to be friends."

"My mother never told me anything about having a conversation with you about my memories."

"Of course, she wouldn't. You think she would want you to know she threatened to destroy our friendship? So, we agreed that I wouldn't ask any more questions about your memory lapse and she wouldn't threaten our friendship."

Neecy stares at Monica for a minute as if she was trying to process the information. "Monica that doesn't mean I've suffered some kind trauma."

"Neecy, then you started having those dreams, you know the ones that someone is choking you. You started having them around the time Miles came into your life."

"Yeah…so?" Neecy does not like where this is going.

"I think Miles asking you questions about your childhood and about your family started to trigger some memories your brain was trying to forget."

"Thanks for saying that in front of Miles. My nightmares where was supposed to stay between you and me."

Miles looks at Neecy. "I knew you were having bad dreams Neecy…I just never said anything."

"What, you knew?"

"Yes. When I heard you whispering and talking to Monica I decided I would wait until you were ready to tell me about them instead of asking you."

"You knew?" Neecy says again staring at Miles.

"Neecy, I was in bed right next to you. How could I not know you were having bad dreams or, should I say, nightmares. I wanted to ask you about them, hold you when you were crying, but you would slip out of bed and call Monica, so I was waiting for you to tell me. That's one of the reasons I've been so protective of you. I am not stalking you or trying to control you, I was trying to protect you."

"Can we stay focused?" Monica interrupts. "You lovebirds can work out all of that later."

"Oh sorry." Neecy and Miles say at the same time.

"As I was saying." continues Monica, "I think Miles asking you all those questions about your childhood and family started to trigger some of the traumatic memories."

"What would the memories have to do with me choking or thinking someone is choking me?" Neecy asks.

"I don't know, that's why I gave you the number to call. It could be anything. Our subconscious compartmentalizes those areas that are too painful to think about until something happens …a trigger occurs and brings it forth."

Miles looked confused, "What do you mean by the trigger?"

Monica explains, "A trigger can be words, ideas, statements, sounds, sights, tastes, or smells that bring up subconscious memories and can set off a strong emotional reaction. They can be conscious or unconscious triggers that go to the depths of pain, frustration, confusion, guilt or shame. Everyone has triggers. The key is being aware of them—what they are about or what caused them—and learning how to manage them instead of them controlling you.

"Triggers aren't always obvious. As a matter of fact, most of the time, they are subtle. That is what keeps you unaware and evokes responses to situations in a certain way. For example, something as simple as hearing a certain tone or sound, or a familiar voice, can bring back specific memories of a time in your life. The memories can be positive or negative. Any time you hear the sound associated with that memory, you are instantly taken back to a specific time in your life or event. Hence you can have dreams, nightmares etc. Unfortunately, left unresolved a person can get stuck in life and continue to relive the traumatic experience, and hence act out accordingly."

"That still doesn't make sense to me Monica." Neecy says. "I hear you, but for some reason, it's not making sense to me."

Monica tells Neecy, "Maybe we should stop for now. After all, you have had a lot thrown at you today."

"No, I need to continue, how does the brain block the memory?"

"Remember, it doesn't happen to everyone in every situation…trauma is subjective. Our conscious mind can only hold 5-9 thoughts at one time. It then does a "data dump" to our subconscious. Our subconscious stores every experience that we have ever had from the moment of conception. It constantly records our experiences, environment, things that are done and said to us and around us. Anything you have ever been exposed to, heard, or seen has been recorded deep within. Those recordings happen through feelings, sight, hearing, smell, and taste. Because our subconscious holds all our life experiences, it also influences our thoughts, actions, and behavior…whether we are aware of it or not.

Monica continues, "Have you ever met someone that you felt you had met before but you couldn't remember where? Have you ever had an experience that frightens you, but you were not sure why? Have you ever wanted to change a behavior or habit and despite your best efforts, you somehow continue the behavior? When information is recorded into the subconscious, it remembers the circumstances. However, it can't distinguish between different situations."

"For example, I was at a conference once and heard a psychologist speaking about a patient she once treated. Her patient was afraid of heights. Not heights in general, only when the patient was high above the ground, and there were no railings or something similar that added extra security. These circumstances would almost send the patient into a full-blown panic attack."

"During a therapy session, the patient had a flash of a baby in a pamper hanging over a tub. Upon further investigation, the patient's mother told him a story about when he was two and she had run some water in the bathtub. When the phone rang, she went to answer it and suddenly heard his older brother screaming. The mother ran back into the bathroom to find the patient's brother hanging on to his diaper. The patient was hanging over the tub with his face in the water. His brother kept him from completely falling in, but he was too small to pull him out. Hence, the patient discovered his fear of heights when there were no barriers or safety precautions to keep him from falling in."

"The subconscious only remembers the fear, the danger, the trauma associated with that event. It's not able to distinguish or gauge the level of danger, or even if the danger is current. Although there may be no conscious memory of the incident, whenever the right circumstances are in place, your subconscious will remember the danger and trigger the fear of the trauma experienced."

"Monica, Miles voice interrupts, maybe we should let Neecy get some rest. Neecy, baby, can I take you home? If you don't want me to stay, I'll leave after I make sure you're settled."

Chapter 11

Make Your Last Breath Count

"Neecy how are you feeling?" Monica asks her best friend.

"I'm numb right now, I don't know what to think. I need time to process everything. We still don't know who this woman is or, at least, we are not sure. I still can't get over how much she looks like me. Her doctor said she is still weak and she has gone back to sleep so no point in hanging around here. I'll come back tomorrow to see if she can talk."

Monica grabs Neecy's hand. "Neecy, I will stay with you, I don't want you to be by yourself right now."

Miles clears his throat, "She's not going to be by herself, I'll be there with her."

"Yeah okay, Jasper...Miles, whoever you are." Monica says in a sarcastic tone. "I don't feel comfortable leaving you alone with my friend."

"If I were going to hurt Neecy, I have had plenty of opportunities to hurt her."

"Can the two of you stop? Both of you can stay. At least something is back to normal with the two of you going back and forth about me. Welcome back."

But first, I want to see my mother." Monica and Miles both stop dead in their tracks.

"See your mother?" Monica frowns. "Neecy sweetie, I don't think that's a good idea."

"I have to see her."

"But baby, her body was burned beyond recognition. I was there. I saw them bring her out."

"You were there?"

Miles shifts his weight and says hesitantly, "Yes, I was there. Angela called and left me a message that she was going over to your mother's house. I was going to meet her, but by the time I got there they were bringing your mother out and the ambulance had already left with her."

"So, her name is Angela?"

"Yeah, Angela McMichael."

"What else do you know that you're not telling me?"

"Neecy, I promise that's all I know. She wouldn't tell me why she wanted to meet your mother before you knew about her. She just kept saying she has to be sure it's you before she tells you who she is, and she kept saying your mother had some explaining do, too. That's all she would say until today when she left the message she was going to your mother's house. She didn't ask me to go with her. Knowing your mother and the tone in Angela's voice, I knew nothing good was about to happen so I headed over to your mother's house, but I was too late."

"Jasper, I mean Miles, you can't beat yourself up about whatever transpired between the two of them...you had no control over that. It sounds like whatever secrets she knows or thinks she knows was already out of anyone's control before she got there. I want her to wake up. I have so many questions, and I'm sure the police do, too."

"Yes they do, my delay in getting there was because I stopped by the police station on my way there."

Neecy and Monica look at Miles, "You stopped by the police station?"

Miles sees their reaction, "I have been a PI for years and a detective before that. I had that feeling a person in my line of work gets when they know a situation isn't going to turn out well. So first I tried to call Detective Sherman. When I couldn't reach him, I stopped by the police station."

"So, you do know more than what you are telling me.

"No Neecy, I don't. Sherm and I go way back. I had asked him to run a background check on Angela. I wanted to find out all I could about her before I exposed her to you. I didn't know she knew where your mother lived, or even who your mother was until she left me that message. I'm not sure how she got your mother's information."

"This whole thing is absolutely bananas and I still need to see my mother."

"Neecy can it wait?"

"No! I have to see her for it to be real to me." Miles and Monica give each other a look, unsure about Neecy's request.

"Neecy, I just don't…"

"I have my mind made up Miles, Jasper, whoever you are.…I'm going to the morgue to see my mother." Now the two of you can come or not, but I'm going." Monica and Miles both know that whenever Neecy announces she has made up her mind, there is no changing it. Monica sighs and Miles says to hold on, let him call Detective Sherman to see where they took the body.

When the three of them arrive at the morgue, Neecy is stone-faced. Monica and Miles are worried about how she will handle seeing an unrecognizable burned body, knowing that it is her mother.

As Neecy walks in, she begins to slow her pace. She can feel her heart racing, as if it's about to jump out her chest. She becomes light-headed but she continues to walk, telling herself she can do this. She thinks to herself, she has to do this. When her father died, he was driving in the mountains, and the car went over a cliff. The police think he committed suicide because there were no skid marks or any signs of him trying to stop the car before it went over the cliff. She didn't get a chance to say goodbye and she never saw his body because they had a closed casket funeral.

The coroner said the body was mangled from the car going over a cliff and rolling multiple times before it came to a stop. Her mother thought it would be too much for her to see the body. Neecy knew she had to say goodbye this time. No one was going to keep her from saying goodbye.

"Hello Ms. Stromm, everyone." the coroner greets them, "Detective Sherman called and told me you were coming. Ma'am, I should warn you, this is highly irregular for the family member to view a body in this condition. We usually confirm ID by dental records or DNA."

"I'm not here to confirm the identity…I have to see her."

"Ma'am the body is badly burned…"

"I don't care." Neecy interrupts the coroner, "I am an emergency room doctor. I've seen it all."

"Okay ma'am, follow me."

Monica and Miles follow Neecy and the coroner down the hall and into a cold room.

"Ma'am, the body is over there, are you ready?"

"Yes, "I'm ready." As Neecy walks toward the body, her knees begin to wobble, Miles catches her just before she hits the ground.

Miles asks, "Neecy are you sure?"

She looks up at him, "Yes, I have to do this." Neecy steadies herself and walks over to the body.

Monica grabs Neecy's hand as the coroner pulls back the sheet. Miles stands behind her in case he needs to catch her again. Neecy stares at the face and then pulls the sheets off the burned body. Her heart is pumping so loud she can't hear any other sounds in the room.

"Where is her necklace?"

"Excuse me ma'am?"

"Where is her necklace? My mother always wore a pendant, she never took it off."

"Ma'am, she didn't come in with one, but that's not unusual. With the heat of the fire and handling of the body, the necklace could have easily fallen off."

"Very well then. Thank you for allowing me to see my mother."

"Monica, Miles, can I have a few minutes alone with my mother? I want to say goodbye."

"Sure Neecy, we will step out. "We will be right outside the door if you need us."

Once out in the hall, Miles looks at Monica, "What do you think?"

"I think she is in shock. We are going to have to keep a close eye on her, even if we have to sleep in shifts. We need to watch her especially since there may be some other trauma we don't know about. We don't know how this is going to impact her until it happens." Monica and Miles begin to whisper so that Neecy won't overhear them planning how they are going to take care of her over the next few days.

Miles suddenly realizes that they have been standing in the hall for a while and asks Monica, "Do you think we should check on her?"

"Yeah, it's been a while since we came out here." Miles eases the door open and softly calls Neecy's name. She doesn't answer. "Neecy." he says again, but Neecy doesn't answer.

"Neecy." Monica calls her name as she approaches her. "Neecy, are you okay? Do you need anything?"

Neecy looks at both of them, turns and walks out the door.

Chapter 12

Whenever I start to feel blue, I start breathing again
~ L. Frank Boum ~

The ride home was quiet. Neecy got lost in her thoughts trying to make sense of the day. Feeling numb and still in disbelief that both her mother and father are gone. She is an only child and doesn't have any family. She wonders to herself how she could feel so alone in this great big world. How can she feel so alone in this moment when Miles and Monica are right there? Maybe this is a dream, and I'm going to wake up any minute. Maybe this is some cruel joke and all will be well in the morning.

Whenever she had a problem she couldn't figure out, her father would tell her to put it out of her mind for the night, sleep on it and all would be well in the morning.

Neecy is startled out of her thoughts when Miles announces they are home. Inside, Neecy notices that somehow her house seems foreign to her. She can't make sense of it. "Do you want me to run you a hot bath baby?"

"No Miles. Thank you, I want to take a shower and lie down."

"Ok, call us if you need anything." Monica announces she is going to fix something light for them to eat...no one had eaten since that morning.

Once inside the bathroom, Neecy turns up the hot water until the bathroom is full of steam. She steps in the shower and starts to remember a song by The Dramatics that her father used to play when her mother was on a rampage. He used to play it over and over in the car when they would drive up to the mountains to get a break from her mother…

> *I wanna go outside in the rain*
> *It may sound crazy*
> *But I wanna go outside, in the rain*
> *Now I, I think I'm gonna cry*
> *Once the rain starts fallin'*
> *On my face (on my face)*
> *You won't see (you won't see, ah)*
> *A single trace (a single trace)*
> *Don't want you to see me cry*
> *Let me go, let me go, let me go*
> *Once the sun comes out*
> *And the rain is gone away*
> *I know I'm going to see a better day…*

As Neecy lets the song play in her head, she lets the water run on her face and imagines that it's raindrops. Then, the pain comes. She starts to feel the pain of the day. It feels as if someone is ripping her heart out of her chest. The grief seems unbearable.

"Oh Lord, you promised me better days. When is the sun coming? When will I see a better day?" She doesn't know how long she had been in the shower or lost in her thoughts when she's startled by a knock on the bathroom door.

"Neecy, it's Monica, are you okay? Dinner is ready if you want to try and eat something. Miles and I will wait for you."

"Okay, I'll be out in a minute." As Neecy joins Monica and Miles at the table, she says, "Thank you guys for being here. I don't think I would have been able to stand the quiet tonight."

"Of course. We are here for you for as long as you need us." Monica says while squeezing Neecy's hand.

"Miles, I know we have some things to work out, but can we put all of that on the back burner for now? I want you here with me if I'm going to get through this. I don't think I can take any other major loss in my life right now."

"Of course baby, whatever you need."

Neecy looks at "Monica…" but Monica cuts her off.

"You know you don't even have to ask, ride or die." Neecy smiles and repeats, "Ride or die."

Neecy starts to laugh uncontrollably. Miles and Monica glance at each other wondering if this is it, if Neecy has reached her breaking point.

Monica asks Neecy what's so funny? "It's funny how things come full circle. Remember the night your father died, I whispered in your ear 'I'm your ride or die,' and this afternoon you reminded me.

Now Monica is laughing too. Miles still looking confused and asked why was ride or die so funny? Neecy explains that when Monica's father died she was distraught, no one could console her. Miles, looking even more confused, asked again how is that funny? Neecy still laughing says "because I whispered in Monica's ear I was her ride or die, but she didn't know what it meant."

Monica, in between laughs, says "Yes, I lived a somewhat sheltered life. Ride or die used to be a biker's old saying. It meant that a biker would rather die than not be able to ride his or her bike. So imagine my confusion when Neecy told me she was my ride or die.

Neecy says, "Yeah and she walked around for weeks expecting me to show up on a motorcycle!"

"But I still didn't know why she thought riding a motorcycle would help me get over my father's death…" They both are now practically on the floor holding their stomachs from laughing so hard.

"I didn't know that she didn't know what it meant. One day she asked me if it was the thrill of the ride on a motorcycle that would help her with her grief." Neecy says, still laughing

By now, Miles has joined them laughing. Neecy says, "I had to explain to her that a ride or die was an idiom. When someone tells you they are your ride or die it means that they will 'ride' out any problems with you or 'die' trying."

At this point, Neecy and Monica are laughing so hard, tears are streaming down their faces. Miles is quite amused and laughs at both of them.

Monica explains, "That's when we agreed that "ride or die" would always be our saying, our signal to each other, especially when life comes to collect what's due. We would always remind the other one that we were each other's ride or die. When tough times come, when life comes to collect what's due, we would get through whatever circumstances came our way together.

Neecy and Monica start laughing again. All of a sudden Monica jumps up and puts on their theme song by Whitney Houston and CeCe Winans, "Count On Me" and starts singing:

> *I can see it's hurting you*
> *I can feel your pain*
> *It's hard to see the sunshine through the rain*
> *I know sometimes it seems as if*
> *It's never gonna end*
> *But you'll get through it*
> *Don't give in because you can*
> *Count on me through thick and thin*
> *A friendship that will never end*

When you are weak, I will be strong
Helping you to carry on
Call on me, I will be there
Don't be afraid
Count on me

As they are holding hands, swaying back and forth, singing loudly and out of tune, Miles begins to see Monica in a different light, from a different perspective. Today he doesn't see her as a busybody friend who can't keep a man and therefore doesn't want her friend to have one. Tonight, he starts to understand their bond, their sisterhood. He begins to see Monica as a loyal friend to Neecy, someone that will "ride or die" to the end, a friend for life. He thinks to himself, "How lucky the two of them are to have that bond between each other. Not everybody is so blessed."

The next thing Miles knows Neecy and Monica are screaming CONCERT!!!!! For the next 30 minutes, Neecy and Monica dance, more like perform every genre of music from country and western songs, to rock and roll, to R&B with dance routines to go with the songs.

Miles is laughing, "Obviously this is not the first time the two of you have gotten together and 'performed.'

"No." Neecy says in between breaths, "when we were kids we used to spend hours learning the verses to our favorite songs, making up dance routines to go with them and then performing them for whoever we could get to be our audience. Karaoke has nothing on us!"

Monica looks over at Miles and nudges Neecy. "Look at how he's looking at you, he has a... CRUSH!!!!" Neecy and Monica yell at the same time. Neecy runs over to her stereo and the next thing Miles knows Neecy and Monica are singing the Avergae White Bands song "School Boy Crush." Neecy circles Miles shaking her finger while singing, "Don't you touch, that ain't much, it's only a schoolboy crush." while Monica pretends to be playing the bass guitar.

Miles clears his throat and reminds them that the food is getting cold. "By the way, can you guys let the professionals sing, and the two of you stick to your day jobs? Neecy and Monica look at each other and grab throw pillows from the couch hitting Miles and chasing him around the room singing Kenny Roger's song "Gambler." "You got to know when to hold 'em, know when to fold 'em, know when to walk away, know when to run." As they double team him, Miles cries out "Uncle" and they all collapse on the floor laughing. As the laughter dies, Neecy begins to look serious again. She looks back and forth sitting between Monica and Miles and tells them both that she loves them.

Monica yells, "GROUP HUG!" As they hug, they go and sit at the table to eat a lukewarm dinner. After dinner, yawning, Neecy announces she's tired and she wants to try and get some rest.

"Monica, you can have the guest room."
"Miles…"

"I know, I'm on the couch. I'll grab a blanket and pillow."

"Miles…" Neecy says looking up at him, "I was going to say you can sleep in my room."

Miles looks at Neecy, "In your room? Together? In the bed together?"

"Yes Miles, in the bed together."

"Alright you two, don't forget you guys have me in the next room. Stay on your respective side of the bed." she says laughing as she walks toward the guest bedroom.

"Neecy, are you sure? I want to be here for you, but I don't want to take advantage of you or the situation."

"Miles, I'm a big girl, I want you to come to bed. Hold me, I need to be held."

"I'll be right there. Just let me check my answering service really quick." Neecy nods and heads to the bedroom as Miles picks up his phone to make the call. "Hey Sherm, this is Miles, any word yet? Ok, call me as soon as you know it's her."

"Miles, how is your girl doing?" asks the detective.

"So far, good. We are just keeping an eye on her." Miles tells him.

"I promise I'll call when I find out anything. You will know when I know."

"Miles…are you coming to bed?" Neecy calls out from the bedroom.

"Hey, I have to go Sherm. I'll give you a call tomorrow."

Chapter 13

Taking Deep Breaths Reduces Tension

Neecy's screams wake Monica. Monica runs into the room and finds Miles and Neecy on the floor.

"What's going on? Why are you on the floor? Neecy are you okay?"

Neecy clings to Miles as Miles explains that Neecy had fallen asleep in his arms. "Once she fell asleep she rolled over on her side of the bed. I fell asleep and woke up to her screaming, squatting over in the corner. I ran over to her and just embraced her where she was...that's when you came in."

"Neecy what's wrong?"

"I don't know Monica. I don't know why I'm in the corner or how I got over here. I remember lying in bed in Jasper's—I mean Miles' arms and waking up over here in the corner with him holding me."

"Baby, can you stand?" asks Miles. Yes, I think so. Miles helps Neecy stand.

"Monica, what's happening to me? Why don't I know why I'm squatting over here in the corner and how I got here?"

"I don't know."

"You don't know? You're the licensed psychologist...what do you mean you don't know?"

Monica takes a deep breath and gives Neecy a stern look. "I don't know for sure, but you may have been sleepwalking."

"Sleepwalking?" Neecy and Miles say at the same time. I've never sleepwalked before...why now?"

"As far as you know, you have never sleepwalked, but it could be all the stress from today's events that caused you to sleepwalk."

"Aye yai yai, so now you're telling me stress made me do it?"

"It's possible, "Neecy, you know how stress works in the body and the negative impact stress can have on the mind and body if it's too much."

Miles looks fascinated. "So Monica, you are telling us that stress can make her ball up in a corner."

"Miles, I'm not saying for sure its stress, but it can be a contributor." "Stress can do all kinds of things to the body."

Miles looks even more intrigued, "Such as?"

"Such as how the body reacts to stress. When you are stressed, your body reacts in a way that is termed 'the fight, flight or freeze response.' It's called the fight, flight or freeze response because internally the subconscious triggers a response that there is danger present. When that trigger happens, your body goes into a natural survival mode to provide the strength and energy to either fight or run away from danger.

"Basically, adrenaline floods into the bloodstream. This, with other stress hormones, causes some changes in your body that are meant to be protective. Your heart rate and blood pressure increase to get more blood to the muscles, brain and heart, you breathe faster to take in more oxygen. Your body prepares for action by tensing your muscles. You're more mentally alert and your sensory organs are heightened to assess the situation and act quickly. Blood flow increases to the brain, heart and muscles, the organs that need it the most. But your skin, digestive tract, kidneys and liver receive less blood because those are the places it is least needed in times of crisis).

There are also things like an increase in blood sugar for extra energy and your body gearing up to prevent hemorrhage in case of injury. These things occur anytime you allow yourself to get stressed out. Your body then absorbs the increased energy because it has no outlet from the buildup.

"Look, stress is natural, but just like anything else, excess stress is unhealthy. It can cause things like significant weight gain or loss, irritability, depression, fatigue, anxiety, anger and the list goes on.

"We experience what I call good stress and bad stress." Monica continues. Like, 'good stress' would be when you're planning for a joyous occasion or event. 'Bad stress' would be when there is a problem or negative situation that has taken a front seat in your life, and you would rather it not be there. Be it good or bad, your body still reacts in the same manner—fight, flight or freeze. When you're physically out of balance, you are mentally and spiritually out of balance.

"Stress is inevitable, the key is learning to manage your stress.

Miles ponders for a minute, "Well, what now?"

Monica looks at Neecy, "Neecy I need for you to call the number I gave you."

"Why can't you do it?"

"Neecy, I've explained to you a thousand times, it would not be ethical for me to take you on as a patient."

"But you already know everything about me." says Neecy.

"Maybe, says Monica, but it would still be unethical. You can be my patient, or you can be my friend. I'm not ready to give up my ride or die, nor do I want to lose you in some other manner, so I need you to call the number I gave you."

"Monica, you know I have trust issues. I don't want to talk to a stranger about any of this."

"If you would call the number and see her, once you get to know her, she won't be a stranger. Neecy please, I'm worried about you. If you can't trust her, then trust me that I wouldn't refer you to someone if I didn't think you'd be in good hands. Promise me you will call in the morning."

"Who are you calling?" asks Miles.

"Monica wants me to call Dr. Megan Goodman. She and Monica went through their Ph.D. program together and studied for their psychologist licenses together. Monica has been trying to get me to go and see her for a couple of years."

"Why haven't you gone?"

"Because my mother was so against it. She didn't want me 'embarrassing' her by going to a shrink."

"Megan is not just any psychologist, "She is a trauma specialist, one of the best in our field, and she's in high demand. She will accept Neecy as a patient as a favor for me. She is just waiting for Neecy to call."

"I think it's a great idea baby."

Neecy frowns, "I don't need to lay on someone's

couch to tell me what's wrong with me. Monica, you already said it's stress."

"I said that stress *could* be contributing and you sound like your mother talking right now. This isn't you Neecy, you're smarter than this."

"Are you saying my mother was dumb?

"No not at all, and we are not even going there, you know that is not what I meant."

"Well, I have made up my mind, Neecy announces, I'm not calling any number. I'm not going to see a head shrink. I've been managing for this long. I will get through this." Miles and Monica look at each other defeated.

"Well, I'm awake now, I want some hot chocolate? Miles, Neecy care to join me?"

"Sure, it's not like I'm going back to sleep anytime soon."

"Miles?"

"No, you two go ahead. I'm going to try to get some sleep. I have to meet with Sherm in the morning."

"You have a meeting with the detective? Does he have an update on my mother's killer?"

"First Neecy, we don't know that anyone killed your mother. And no, I was working on another case. He called and said he has some information for me. I shouldn't be gone long. In fact, you two will probably still be asleep by the time I return." Mile's says as he heads toward the bedroom.

"Neecy, you are out of hot chocolate…do you want some coffee?"

"No thanks, I think I'm going to try and get some sleep. I have been up for the past two days."

"The past two days?"

"Yes, so much has happened in the past two days. We haven't had a chance to talk. I went up to the mountains and Miles followed me."

"What do you mean followed you?"

"We were arguing, I walked out, and he followed me. I didn't know he had followed me up to my cabin until the next morning."

"Ohhh, that's why you weren't returning my phone calls." Monica says. "You don't get reception up there."

"Yes, I just wanted to get away, to clear my head. Monica, can we talk about this later, I'm tired?"

"Of course." Monica says with a yawn, "I'm going to go back to bed too."

Chapter 14

To Be A Christian Without Prayer Is No More Possible
Than To Be Alive Without Breathing
~ Martin Luther ~

"Where is she? I've been calling and leaving messages on her cell phone. I even started leaving messages at the hotel where she said she was staying. It's been five days…I pray nothing has happened to her. If something were to happen to my PattyCake, I don't think I could stand it. My old heart couldn't take it."

As Patty paces up and down the floor, she prays out loud, "Oh, Lord, my strength and my redeemer. I don't ask for much Lord, but please hear my prayer. Please Lord, watch over my PattyCake, let her be alright. I can't lose her too Lord. Lord you know the pain this family has been through. After all this time, you can't take my PattyCake away from us too. I don't think this family can make it through another loss."

"Lord, I ask that you cover her and keep her, and for whatever reason she is not answering her phone, let her be alright. I pray this prayer as humble as I know how Lord. I ask that you let her be okay and that you allow her to come back to us Lord. Please PattyCake, please be okay. My heart can't take the pain of losing you. I'm worried sick about you. Lord, please let her call and say she is okay."

"Well hello Ma'am, you gave us quite a scare. There were a lot of people praying for you if you believe in that sort of thing. How are you feeling this morning?"

Angela is looking around the room, thinking to herself this looks like a hospital room and the lady talking to her is dressed in scrubs. Am I dreaming? The last thing I remember was calling Miles. Angela looks over at the nurse and asks, "Where am I?"

"Ma'am, you're in the hospital."

"Hospital?" Angela tries to sit up.

"Ma'am, I don't think you should try to get up, you have some pretty serious injuries. It was touch and go for a moment. We weren't sure you were going to pull through."

"Touch and go? Hospital? What happened?"

"Ma'am, do you know your name?"

"Of course, I know my name. My name is Angela, Angela McMichael."

"Okay, Ms. McMichael, hold on. I'm going to call the doctor for you."

"Nurse can you tell me what happened?" Angela asks.

"I'm going to get the doctor for you to answer your questions."

Angela thinks to herself and tries to remember the day's events, but all she can remember is calling Miles. How did she end up in the hospital? "My head feels like a Mack truck ran over it and my side hurts." Angela reaches for her side and feels the bandages. She tries to sit up again, horrified at the feel of the bandages.

"Ma'am we can't let you get up just yet. We have to wait for the doctor to examine you...he is on his way. Angela continues to struggle and keeps trying to sit up, trying to speak but the words won't come.

"Ma'am if you keep trying to get out of bed, we will have to restrain you."

"Restraints?" Angela manages to get out.

"Yes, restrain you. You have some pretty serious injuries and you need to stay in bed."

"Hello Ms. McMichael, I'm Dr. Turner. You gave us a quite a scare." Angela looks confused.

"Doctor can you tell me what happened, how did I end up in the hospital? What are these bandages?"

"Ms. McMichael, you were in a house fire. You were brought in an ambulance with bruising on your face, a stab wound, and smoke inhalation."

"Fire, stabbed…what? None of this makes sense, I don't remember any of this. Where is Miles?"

"Who ma'am?"

"Miles, he was here."

Dr. Turner looks at the nurse and the nurse whispers that no one has been there today. Dr. Turner turns back to Angela, "Ma'am, no one has been here today."

"Yes, he was here, he was talking to me. He was here with some other people. I heard them talking, but I didn't recognize anyone's voice but Miles. Where is he?"

The nurse leans towards Angela, "Ma'am no one has been here today. There's a gentleman that has stopped by every day since you've been here, but he hasn't been here today."

"What do you mean he has stopped by every day? How long have I been here? What day is it?"

"Ma'am, you were admitted to the hospital five days ago. You have been drifting in and out of consciousness."

"What? Five days ago? How is that possible? Someone, please find Miles! I have to get out of here…she might be in danger." Angela throws the covers back and tries to sit up.

Dr. Turner tells the nurse to get the restraints. As the nurses are strapping her in, one of them tells her it's for her safety. "Once you calm down, we will remove the restraints."

"Find Miles! Someone, please find Miles!"

Dr. Turner tells Angela he needs her to calm down so that he can finish examining her.

"I don't want to calm down. "Don't you understand…she may be in danger! I have to find her. I need to talk to Miles."

"Danger? Who is in danger Ms. McMichael?"

"*She's* in danger…I need to talk to Miles."

Dr. Turner is thinking to himself how much she looks like Neecy. He can't believe the resemblance and thinks to himself they have to be related.

"Ms. McMichael, do you remember anything else about that day? How you got hurt?"

"No, no I don't. Doctor, why can't I remember?"

Dr. Turner explains that when trauma occurs, the front part of our brain shuts down, and the brain recording mechanism can stop memories from being properly stored. In some cases, the part of our brain that stores our long-term memory is suppressed and either the memory of the event isn't stored, or it is stored but because of the effects on the brain, it's difficult to recall memories.

"However." he continues, "we do know that the memories can be recalled with rest which allows the brain to heal."

"So, you're telling me I will be able to remember what happened if I rest?"

"Let me just say, it's possible. It doesn't always happen. Sometimes memories of a traumatic event are lost forever, but the sooner the person is stabilized and allowed to rest, it increases the possibility of recall."

"I don't have time to rest, I need to know what's happening." Angela struggles with the restraints again.

Dr. Turner turns to the nurse, "Nurse call me when she calms down. Also give Dr. Stromm and Detective Sherman a call and let them know she is awake. Ms. McMichael, I am going to finish my rounds and I will come back to check on you a little later."

By now Angela has drifted into her thoughts. "Why can't I remember what happened? I've been here five days? Hopefully Miles will be able to make sense of all this. I hope she is ok, I remember calling Miles to tell him I was on my way over to her mother's house. Why can't I remember more? If I've been here five days, everybody must be in a panic looking for me, especially Mama Patty. Mama is the only one that knows I was coming here and why. She must be worried sick. I need a phone, uuhh, I forgot I was in these restraints. I can't move. "Nurse, is anyone out there, Nurse!"

Chapter 15

Holding Your Breath Creates The Urge To Breathe

"Yes Ms. McMichael, what can I get for you?"

"Nurse, I need to use the phone, my family doesn't know I'm here."

"If you give me the name and phone number, I can call them for you."

"No, I need to call my mother myself. I'm sure by now she is a basket case and she won't be okay until she hears my voice."

Okay, Ms. McMichael, I'm going to loosen the restraints. Don't make me regret it. You can use my cell phone, but don't tell anyone I let you use it…I could get fired. It's our secret."

"Absolutely, it's our secret. Thank you."

"Hello Mama, it's me, Angela."

"PattyCake! Is that you! Thank you Jesus! Thank you, Lord! Thank the Lord…He answered my prayers. PattyCake, where are you? Are you okay?"

"Yes and no. Yes, I'm okay, but I am in the hospital."

"Hospital! For what? What's wrong? What happened!"

"It's a long story Mama and I'm not quite sure myself."

"What do you mean you're not sure what happened?"

"Just what I said. I can't remember what happened. I woke up in the hospital today with bandages."

"Bandages, what kind of bandages?

"The doctor says someone stabbed me."

"STABBED! Oh my Lord! I knew I shouldn't have let you go by yourself."

"It's not your fault Mama. Remember I took a leave of absence from my practice because I didn't know how long I would need to be here."

"Did she hurt you, was it her?" "I can't remember Mama. All I can remember is that I was headed to her house." "If she hurt my PattyCake the saying hell has no fury won't have anything on me. That woman will feel my wrath like she has never felt anyone's wrath before."

"Mama, I need for you to calm down. The doctor said I should make a full recovery and hopefully remember what happened."

"PattyCake, what hospital are you in? Mama Patty is on her way."

"Yes, Ma'am. I'm going to hand the phone to my nurse and she will be able to give you the information. Mama, can you bring the envelope with you. And Mama, can you hurry? I'm scared."

"Don't you worry 'bout nothing PattyCake. I'm on my way. Let me talk to that nurse."

Patty thanks the nurse, hangs up the phone and starts crying. "Thank you Lord for watching over my PattyCake. Thank you Jesus for hearing my prayers. Lord, I ask that you watch over me in my travels as I catch this plane to see about my PattyCake.

"And Lord, if that woman has hurt my PattyCake, if she is responsible for hurting one hair on her head, she is gonna have to deal with me. Now Lord, you know I'm a saved woman. Lord you know I'm not a violent woman. I don't want to have to lay my religion down, but this woman has already brought too much pain to this family. I mean it Lord…your child can only take so much. So Lord, I ask that you help me hold my peace until I know what happened, but if she has hurt my baby, I can't promise you what I will or won't do. Amen!"

The nurse looks at Angela and asks if she needs anything else. Angela asks for some water and thanks the nurse again for letting her use her phone.

"No problem Ms. McMichael, I wouldn't want my family worrying about me. Ms. McMichael, I have a question, may I ask why your mother called you PattyCake?"

Angela starts to smile, "Oh yes, my mother has called me PattyCake since I was a little girl, for as long as I can remember. And she is so protective of the name, no one else in the family can call me PattyCake. She said it's just a name for her. I am her PattyCake."

"Please don't ask me what it means, or how she came to call me that. It's just one of those things that happen in a family…when the family gives you a nickname and it sticks." she says laughing.

The nurse smiles, "It's such a strong term of endearment. I just wondered. I hope you didn't mind me asking."

"No, not at all."

"It sounds like the two of you are close?"

"Yes, thicker than thieves."

"I better quit being nosy and let you get some rest while I check on my other patients. Here is the call button if you need anything. Push this button for the nurse's station and someone will come and see about you."

"Thank you, Nurse."

Angela tries to get comfortable and starts to go over the sequence of events in her head hoping that it will help trigger her memory of what happened. Let's see, I remember Miles giving me an update on the possibility of finding Neecy. Then I jumped on the computer and Googled her name. Once I saw the picture, I knew it had to be her. I remember trying to call Mama Patty but she didn't answer the phone. I didn't leave a message…I just figured it was probably best that I didn't tell Mama I found her until I knew for sure.

What also came up in the Google search was Shanice and a picture of her mother with their address. That's when I called Miles back and told him I was going over there. He told me to wait for him, so I waited an hour but I couldn't wait any longer. When I called him back, it went straight to voicemail, so I left a message for him to meet me there.

I jumped in the rental car, put the address in the GPS and headed to her house. On my way there I called Miles again, and this time he answered. I told him I was going over there, and he told me he didn't think it was a good idea. I thanked him for his concern and his services and told him I would take it from here. He told me he didn't think it was a good idea that I go to her house alone because it could be dangerous, so he would meet me there. I told him not to be ridiculous…what could happen?

He told me he had learned some new information he had not had a chance to share with me and that he was on his way. I remember parking a block away because I didn't want her to know what kind of car I was driving. Why can't I remember what happened beyond that? Not knowing what happened is driving me crazy. My memory has to come back and come back soon.

I hope Mama can get here soon. She knows how much I hate hospitals. It's been that way since I was a child. I don't know why…I have just never been able to stand the smell, the energy of a hospital. Mama Patty has always been there for me. She took me in when I had no place to go and raised me as her own. What I most admire about her is that she would never let me call her Mama. She always said it felt like it would be dishonoring my mother even though she loves me as her own. My Mama Patty is my strength and the pillar of the family. Her faith in God is what I think keeps her going. I'm thirsty, where is that call button?"

Chapter 16

Breathe In, Breathe Out

"My mother didn't have a lot of friends and she didn't have any family. That leaves just a couple of people that lived on the block and a few people that she worked with to notify about her memorial service. She wanted to be cremated, so we don't have to worry about selecting a grave site. I have to find a place to hold the memorial services. I'm looking for a nice picture of her...that was another quirk with my mother, she didn't like taking pictures." Neecy starts to cry again. Her eyes already swollen and red, Monica hugs her and tells her she will get through this. Neecy nods. "I know, losing her is so painful. I didn't ever want to feel this pain again after my father died."

"I used to ask God to take me before you or my mother because I didn't ever want to feel this kind of pain again."

"Neecy, I never knew that."

"Yeah, you know I don't handle these kinds of situations well when it affects me personally. Isn't it funny how I work in an emergency room, see people die all the time, families distraught, but it doesn't have a major impact on me? I don't fall to pieces when I lose a patient. Don't get me wrong, I'm sad when I have to tell them that their loved one didn't make it, but I don't fall to pieces."

"That's because you have become desensitized to other's loss…we both suppress our feelings. It's a defense mechanism, and that's a good thing. We have to make sure our concern for our patient's pain doesn't distract us from the task at hand. If we didn't, we would be basket cases carrying all that sadness and depressive energy. The time to become concerned is when you don't feel anything, or if everything affects us to the point that we can't do our jobs."

"Neecy is that your phone ringing?"

"Yes, I left it in the bedroom, hold that thought."

"Hello Dr. Stromm, this is the nurse's station. You asked that we give you a call when the patient awakens."

"How long has she been awake?"

"Since yesterday Doctor, there was an error when she was transferred from ICU to a regular room. We didn't see the note until just now with the instructions to call you when she was awake. Hello… Dr. Stromm?"

Neecy is so anxious to get to the hospital, she hangs up the phone without saying goodbye to the nurse. Monica is sitting at the table helping Neecy go over the funeral arrangements, she looks up at Neecy, what's up?

"She's awake." Neecy says as she grabs her keys.

"Hold on Neecy, I'll drive. I want us to get there in one piece. You can call Miles on the way and let him know where we are going to the hospital." Neecy nods and tosses Monica the keys.

"I want to know what she did to my mother and why? Why did she set the house on fire?"

"Now Neecy, we don't know what happened."

"Don't tell me you are taking Miles' side."

"I'm not taking anybody's side. I think we should wait to hear what she has to say and what the investigation yields."

"What other explanation can there be Monica? This woman is at mother's house, there is a fire, and my mother is burned beyond recognition. What can she possibly say?"

"Neecy, you need to remain calm when we get to the hospital, or you may never know. Promise me you won't start the conversation with accusations."

"I can't promise that Monica."

"Okay, then let me start the conversation. In fact, let me do all the talking, and hopefully we can get some answers."

When Neecy and Monica arrive at the woman's room, Detective Sherman is walking out. "Detective, did you find out why she killed my mother? Is she under arrest?" Detective Sherman shakes his head, "No Ma'am, we are still investigating. We must verify her story."

"What story? What is she telling you happened?"

"Ma'am, I can't provide any information yet because it's an ongoing investigation, but as soon as I'm able talk to you, I will tell you everything I can."

"That's not good enough, Detective. Somebody is going to tell me why she hurt my mother. If you don't tell me today, she will." Neecy says pointing at the woman's room.

"Neecy, we agreed that you wouldn't walk in making accusations."

"No Monica, you agreed. I didn't agree to anything." Neecy says, walking toward the woman's room. Monica and Detective Sherman follow her.

As Neecy approaches the woman's bed, she is again taken aback by how much they look alike and now that some of the swelling in her face has gone down, she thinks to herself they look so much alike they could be twins. Angela has her eyes closed and doesn't see Neecy approaching her. As soon as she senses someone in the room, her eyes pop open. Her and Neecy stare at each other, both at a loss for words. Monica and the detective are staring back and forth also at a loss for words because of the resemblance. After a few minutes of silence, Neecy finally manages to ask, "What's your name?"

"PattyCake, is that you PattyCake? Oh, dear Jesus, thank God… you are okay. I didn't know what I would find when I got here. I'm here now PattyCake, Mama Patty is here to take care of you." Angela looks past Neecy to the sound of Patty's voice coming toward her. "Mama, I'm so glad you are here. I'm sorry I didn't listen."

"Don't you worry about a thing PattyCake. You have nothing to be sorry about, and if that woman hurt you, she will be sorry." Neecy steps toward Patty, "Are you talking about my mother?"

Mama Patty turns toward Neecy, half startled because she was so focused on Angela she didn't even notice Neecy, Monica or the detective standing in the room. When she looks at Neecy, she starts screaming "Oh my God! Oh, Dear Sweet Jesus! I can't believe it! Sweet Jesus!" Patty starts to feel the blood rushing to her head as Detective Sherman reaches out and grabs her before she hits the floor. Monica grabs a chair and Detective Sherman helps Patty ease into the chair.

Patty slowly looks Neecy up and down, then looks at Angela and looks back at Neecy. All she can manage to say is "Sweet Jesus!" Patty starts to hyperventilate.

"Ma'am, I'm going to help you slow down your breathing before you pass out. Now take a deep breath with me. That's it, blow it out slowly. Take another deep breath, slow it down, now breath it out slowly. Breath with me, in, out, that's it." As Monica continues to help Patty breathe, Angela is trying to sit up. Neecy takes the control and raises her head on the bed.

Monica tells Mama Patty to continue to breathe, as she backs away. Monica and Detective Sherman are now standing looking back and forth at the three of them. Monica is speechless and thinks to herself, they have to be related, cousins or something. Detective Sherman is also lost in his thoughts. "This case is getting more interesting by the minute. I can't wait to put the pieces of this puzzle together."

Neecy finally asks, "Who are you people?" Still saying Sweet Jesus, Patty jumps out of her chair and tries to hug Neecy. Neecy backs away, not sure how she should respond to Patty's attempt to hug her. Neecy repeats, "Who are you people?"

"Chile', I'm your Aunt Patty." Angela touches Patty's arm and reminds her about the letter and that she doesn't know. Neecy looks confused, "I don't know what?"

Angela clears her throat and tries to adjust to her bed, but suddenly looks past Neecy and says, "Miles, thank you for coming." Everyone turns to see Miles walking in the room. Miles walks over to Angela's bed and tells her he is glad she is alright. Neecy now, clearly irritated, looks from Miles to Angela to Patty and back to Miles. "Somebody better start explaining before I get upset."

Just at the moment Miles is about to speak, the nurse comes in and informs them that there are too many people in the room. Visiting hours are over and everyone has to leave. Patty quickly says she is not going anywhere. As long as Angela is in the hospital that is where she will be. The nurse nods and announces to the room that everyone else has to leave, "Ms. McMichael's needs her rest."

"I can't leave now, I need some answers."

"Neecy, we better go." Monica says. "We know the hospital rules better than anyone. Besides, we need to finish planning your mother's memorial service. And Neecy, you need to rest too." Outside the room, everyone agrees to meet tomorrow morning in Angela's room.

Chapter 17

Exhilaration Is Sharing A Breath

The sun is shining so bright it wakes Neecy. As she rubs the sleep from her eyes, she rolls over to check the time. "Oh my God! It's almost noon! We were supposed to meet at the hospital at noon!" Neecy runs out of the room and sees Miles and Monica sitting at the table. "Why didn't someone wake me?"

"Calm down baby." Miles says.

"Don't tell me to calm down…why didn't you wake me? I have to get ready to go to the hospital."

"You were sleeping. This is the first time since all this started that you slept through the night without waking up screaming or squatting in the corner crying. We wanted you to be able to sleep for as long as you could."

"Well, I'm awake now, I'm going to get ready to go to the hospital."

"Neecy clam down she's not there." "What do you mean she is not there?" "Sherm called me this morning from the hospital, he went up earlier than the time we set because he wanted to ask Angela some questions about his investigation before we got there. He said when he got there the nurse informed him that Angela had already been discharged from the hospital." "Discharged? Where did they go, back to her hotel? Let's go to her hotel."

"She's not there".

"What do you mean she's not there, where can she be?"

"We don't know. At least she is not staying at the hotel she was at before all of this happened."

Neecy raises an eyebrow, and how do you know where she was staying Miles?"

"She told me when she flew here to meet you."

Neecy rolls her eyes, "Does anyone know where her mother is staying?"

"No, we don't have any info right now. Sherm is trying to track them down as we speak, so all we can do is wait. Wait, this woman shows up, my mother is dead, her mother claims to be related to me, to be my aunt and now I'm supposed just to wait?"

"Neecy, what else is there to do but wait?"

Neecy sighs. "There was something I thought about last night when I was drifting off to sleep. Sometimes I have this dream that I hadn't thought about in a long time. The dream is me as a little girl. In the dreams I'm playing with another girl that is dressed like me and we look alike. We always have on a striped red shirt and some denim shorts with white sneakers. I thought maybe it was a symbolic dream, one of those types of dreams you have when you're wrestling with a decision and seeing yourself in your own dream. I never thought much of it until now. Monica, what do you think it means?"

"Neecy, I'm reluctant to give any interpretation or opinions right now. There are so many unanswered questions, but I definitely think it has something to do with Angela showing up."

"I don't know, I need answers."

Miles puts his arm around Neecy, "I know and you will have them. Angela hired me to find you. Once I found you, she flew here to meet you and now her mother is here. They haven't gone through all this trouble to find you to just pick up and leave. They aren't going anywhere until they talk to you. But for now, we need to go over to the funeral home to finalize things for your mother's memorial service tomorrow."

"I would like for both of you to go with me."

"Of course we are going." Miles says as he squeezes her shoulder.

"I still can't believe she is gone" as the tears start to sting her eyes.

Neecy drifts into thoughts about her mother. Neecy loved her mother, but she was never extremely close to Alice. They didn't have a mother-daughter bond as she has witnessed with other mothers and daughters. For instance, Monica and her mother are extremely close...you can see and feel the bond they share when you are around them. Neecy thinks my mother and I never had that kind of bond. There always seemed to be this distance between us that she couldn't figure out. Sometimes Neecy even felt as if she stayed in touch with her out of an unspoken loyalty required between a daughter and her mother. Especially after Neecy's father died, Alice seemed to become even more distant and guarded. Neecy thinks to herself, "None of this matters now...she's gone."

Chapter 18

Shallow Breaths Count As Breathing

"Mama, thank you for being here.

"Nonsense, you never have to thank me. Where else would I be? Since the doctor has not cleared you to travel and the police don't want you to leave town, I moved us to this hotel with a suite so that you can recover more comfortably."

"Thanks, Mama."

"You get some rest PattyCake. I'm going to go over to the hotel you were staying to get your things. You might as well get comfortable...it looks like we are going to be here for a while. Here, let me help you get in bed."

As Angela gets into bed, she smiles at Patty. "Mama, can you believe we found her? We found her alive and well? I've been praying for this day, ever since the letter showed up. I have been praying that we would find her alive and well. The Lord has answered our prayers."

"I still thank my Lord and Savior, but God this has been possible. I'm sorry I got so excited and blurted out I was her aunt, it just happened." "I know Mama, but don't worry."

"I'm sure she has questions, and there doesn't appear to be any damage done."

"I hope not, I would never forgive myself to know that we were so close, to only lose her again."

"We are not going to lose her. I believe everything happens for a reason, when it is supposed to happen. Sometimes we have to trust that everything will happen in its time. We have waited this long, it won't hurt to wait a few more days."

"I need to get some rest and more strength before we talk to her."

"I agree PattyCake, you always did have the patience of Job. I'm just excited and can't wait for her to know the truth, that we are her family."

"We have to keep in mind, Mama, that our truth may be a tragedy for her. That's why the letter warned us to be careful in our approach with her. I know, and I will follow your lead from now on, especially when we talk to her. Now get some rest, I'm going to run out for a few minutes and take care of some things".

"If you get hungry before I get back, just order room service." says Patty as she heads toward the door. "I will also stop at the store and pick up a few things for dinner. Do you need anything PattyCake?"

"No, I'm just going to sleep, I still don't have 100% of my energy back."

"The doctor said you lost a lot of blood. Because of your injury, he said it could be a few more days before you felt like getting out and about. Sleep PattyCake, the body heals faster when you sleep." I'm going to put the Do Not Disturb sign on the door so that the maid doesn't come in and disturb you while I'm gone."

"Lord, it's me again, Patty. These children have been through so much. These are the times that I have to trust that you know what you are doing, that there is a purpose for all of this. Lord, I ask that you give me the wisdom to know what to say and when to say it. Lord help us get through this. Thank you for letting us find her. I ask that you continue to watch over us all. Amen."

"Now, what did I do with those keys and my grocery list?"

As Patty is pulling out into the traffic, Detective Sherman is pulling into the hotel parking lot, they miss each other. He wonders to himself if he should have called first and scheduled a time to talk. But the element of surprise is sometimes better. The first 48 hours of a crime is crucial, and he has already lost days of what could be key information about what happened.

"Who is banging on this door?" Mama must have forgotten her room key or forgot to put the do not disturb sign on the door. "It's going to take me a few minutes to get up. I'm feeling better, but I still have some pain if I try to move too fast."

"Who is it?" Angela yells through the door.

"Ma'am, it's Detective Sherman."

Angela takes a deep breath and opens the door.

"Yes Detective, how can I help you?"

"Ma'am is it okay for me to come in? I have some follow up questions about the investigation."

"Sure, come in." Angela says opening the door wider for him to enter.

"Ma'am, how are you feeling?" Detective Sherman asks.

"I'm getting better by the day."

"Is it okay if I ask you some more questions?"

"You can ask, but I can't say that I remember anything else."

"Ma'am, in my experience, it helps to talk through the sequence of events. Sometimes the details of what happened are easier to remember while you talk through what happened. People tend to recall details they previously forgot."

"Okay, I'll try. What is it you want to know?"

"Can you tell me again what happened, starting from when you drove over to the house and parked the car?"

As Angela replays the sequence of events in her head, she suddenly becomes excited. "I remember walking up to the door and knocking. That woman opened the door. At first she must have thought I was Neecy because when she opened the door, she asked me why I didn't use my key.

When I said I have never had a key, she looked at me startled, as if she had seen a ghost. She asked me what I wanted, why was I there. I responded and told her I think she knows, and she signaled for me to come in and sit down. She said, I knew this day would come, I should have followed my first instinct years ago."

"Ma'am, what did she mean by that?"

"I'm not sure, she didn't elaborate."

Detective Sherman continues his line of questioning, "What happened next?"

"I remember telling her I was there to see Neecy, I just had to make sure it was her before I approached Neecy. She laughed and asked me if I thought she was about to let that happen."

"I told her it wasn't her choice, I have the letter, and I know everything. At that point, she got unusually calm, eerie calm, and asked me if I was hungry or wanted some tea. I felt this chill go up my spine and told her I needed to leave. She told me, nonsense, and that I seemed like a reasonable woman. 'Let's talk about why you are here,' she said. 'There must be a way this could be a win-win for everybody.' I should have followed my instincts and left, but instead I followed her into the kitchen."

"Do you know what she meant by that ma'am, that it could be a win-win for everybody?"

"No, we never had the conversation. She rinsed out a tea kettle and turned the fire up on the stove.

Things happened so fast after that…it's all a blur. The next thing I know she was coming at me with a knife, murmuring something about I must be crazy and how easy it will be to convince the police that I attacked her. We started struggling over the knife and suddenly, I felt a sharp pain."

"I fell to the ground, but I knew I couldn't stop fighting her or she would kill me. As she tried to stab me again, somehow I was able to kick her and she fell back on the stove. I remember hearing her scream out. I'm not sure if she burned herself or if she fell on the knife because at that point, I was lying on the floor fighting to stay conscious."

"I remember thinking, I have to make sure she is not continuing to try and hurt me. I forced my eyes open in time to see a large flame. At that point, I wasn't sure if I was still conscious or dreaming. She tried to run past me. I remember grabbing her leg and she fell next to me. She was screaming that the kitchen was on fire, and to let her go before we both died in there. At that point, I must have passed out because I don't remember anything else until I woke up in the hospital."

"That chick better be glad I don't cuss and she better be especially glad that she is already dead!" Detective Sherman and Angela turn to see Patty standing behind them.

"Mama! How much did you hear?"

"I heard it all. I saw Detective Sherman pulling into the hotel parking lot when I was pulling into traffic so I circled the block and came back. I didn't interrupt because I didn't know if it would cause you to lose your thoughts."

"Ma'am, would you like to join us?"

"Yes, PattyCake, is that okay with you?"

"Yes, Mama, of course you can join us. I'm glad you came back." Patty sits next to Angela.

"Ma'am is there anything else you remember?"

"Not right now."

"PattyCake, did you tell him about the letter?"

"Thanks, Ma'am, I was going to circle back to that. Ma'am, you mentioned a letter, you have a letter?"

Angela takes a deep breath and readjusts how she is sitting as if she was trying to get comfortable.

"PattyCake are you ok? Is this too much?"

"No Mama, I want to get this out and give Detective Sherman all the information we have."

"Thank you Ma'am, but only if you feel up to it. Can you tell me about the letter?" Angela nods her head and takes another deep breath. "About a year ago, a letter was mailed to my business address."

"What do you do Ma'am?" asks Detective Sherman. "I'm an attorney." Detective Sherman writes something and then looks up from his pad, ma'am, please continue.

"About a year ago, a letter was mailed to my practice with no return address. The envelope looked old, as if it had been kept for a long time. "What did the letter say?" "It was a letter from my father, or at least someone claiming to be my father." At that point, Angela and Patty could feel the tears stinging their eyes.

"Why do you say 'claiming to be your father?'"

"Because up until that time, I thought…my family thought that he and my mother had died in a house fire when I was six years old."

Patty reaches for a tissue and hands Angela one. "My father's body was never recovered because the house exploded due to the gas leaking. The cause of death was determined to be death by explosion. They were able to recover my mother's body because she was in a different part of the house. Once the autopsy was completed, the coroner ruled it a homicide because my mother had been stabbed."

"What does your father's death have to do with the letter you received and with you going to see Ms. Stromm?" Angela reaches for another tissue. "The letter started off with, 'If you are reading this, I am dead or will be by the time this reaches you. My father went on to explain what happened the day of the fire. He explains in the letter that he didn't die in the fire. He had been in hiding all these years and that he was sorry for everything that happened. He explained that he and my mother were not getting along, they had separated for a short time and filed for divorce. "

"During the time they were separated, he met another woman and had an affair. After he started seeing the other woman he and my mother had decided to give their marriage another try, so he tried to end the affair. He shared in the letter that my mother knew about the other woman but was willing to forgive him because he had not started the affair until after they had separated and filed for divorce. He said the woman he was having an affair with was named Alice Johnston—"

"Which you think is Alice Stromm?"

"Not think, I know. My father had enclosed a picture of her in the letter that was sent to me. It was a young version of her, but it was definitely her."

"The letter said that when he tried to end the affair, Alice went ballistic, started calling the house, driving by, threatening to call my mother. When she found out my mother already knew about her, she showed up at the house one day, the day my mother died." Angela and Patty are crying, and Patty asked Angela how she was feeling. Angela wipes her nose and looks at Detective Sherman. "I'm sorry, I thought I could do this, but I just can't right now. Can we take a break?"

"Yes, of course, would it be okay if I come back tomorrow?"

"Yes, that's fine. I just want to lie down right now, my eyelids are so heavy, and I'm drained."

"Thank you, Ma'am, for taking the time to speak with me. What time would you like for me to stop by tomorrow, and only if you are up to it?"

"This time tomorrow will be fine."

"Tomorrow it is. I'm sorry for your loss." As he is walking to the door, Sherm is deep in thought about the story he just heard. He thinks to himself, "...and the plot thickens." He bids goodbye to the ladies again before turning to walk out. He reminds them to call him if they have any questions or if they need anything he can assist with.

Patty helps Angela back to bed. "Mama? Yes baby? Can we call Neecy tomorrow? I'm anxious to talk to her."

"Yes, baby, I will call her in the morning. In the meantime, you get some rest, and I'm going to head back out to finish my errands. Are you hungry? Do you want me to order room service?" Angela doesn't answer because she has already drifted off to sleep.

Chapter 19

Breathing Is A Sign Of Life

"The funeral home has done a nice job." Monica says looking around. "Where did you find that picture of your mother, Neecy?"

"Among some of my old college stuff. Last night I remembered she let me take it when I was home one year for summer break. She was a beautiful lady. I still can't believe she is gone…this all seems so unreal."

"Well, maybe the services in the morning will help you start to wrap your mind around it." says Monica.

"I hope so. Even though I've been crying, I don't think it has sunk in yet that she is gone."

Monica smiles at Neecy and hugs her. "Where did Miles go?" Neecy asks. "He stepped out to take a call when you were in the bathroom. He said he is working on a case and was trying to tie up some loose ends. He should be back any minute… I know he doesn't like leaving your side."

"You know Neecy, I have to admit, I may have been wrong about Miles. Watching him over the last few days, it's apparent that he cares about you."

"I don't know if I necessarily agree with the stalking tendencies, but the more of what's revealed about what's going on, he may have good reasons for wanting to stay close to you at all times."

"Thanks for saying that Monica, but I have more issues with Miles and our relationship than I did before the recent events occurred. Not to mention, he lied to me not only about who he is, but about everything. I don't know if we are going to be able to work through it. How can I trust him after all of this? I love him but trusting him is going to be a different story. As I already told him, I just can't deal with another loss right now. I do need him right now, so that's why I put us on the back burner, but I will have to address my issues with him. He's not off the hook."

"I hear you, and I think it's smart that you are not trying to deal with relationship issues while everything else is going on. Whatever you decide, you know I will support you."

"Have you decided what you are going to do with the ashes?"

"No, with the exception of her mentioning she wanted to be cremated, my mother and I never had a conversation about if she died. In fact, whenever I tried to bring it up, she would laugh and say she is going to live forever and change the subject."

Monica sighs, "She could be a little arrogant at times, and somewhat over the top, even grandiose."

"Monica, how can you say that about the dead?"

"It would be inappropriate to make up things about your mother, but we both know it's true."

"I know, and she definitely had some demons in her closet that seemed to haunt her. She would never talk about her past or how she was brought up in foster homes, so I have no idea what demons she was dealing with. I just assumed that growing up the way she did caused her to be rough around the edges, sometimes even prickly."

"Changing the subject, when do you think we will hear from Angela and her mother?"

"I don't know. Like Miles said, all we can do is wait. I agree with him—they have gone through too much to find you to leave without contacting you. Neecy, I haven't said anything until now, but I have to ask, is it possible you are related to them? All of you do look remarkably alike."

"I've been thinking about that myself. It's possible. I know my father had family out there somewhere, but because he lost contact years ago and never talked about them, I don't know anything about them. It's no coincidence how much Angela and I look alike. It's possible we are related, cousins maybe."

"Thanks for the update Sherm." Miles is outside talking on the phone. "Do you think she is credible? Did she say anything about seeing Neecy? Neecy is anxious to talk to them. Once her mother's memorial services are over, there won't be any distractions. Trust, if I know my lady, her full attention will be focused on talking to them. So let me know when you think she has her strength back and can see us. We are at the funeral home now. I stepped outside to take your call, so I better get back in there before Neecy starts to get suspicious. I'll call you later."

"There you two are." says Miles as he walks back inside.

"Were you able to take care of your business?" Neecy asks Miles looking up at him. "Yes, somewhat. "How are *you* doing baby…do you need anything?" "No Miles, not right now, I'm glad both of you are here."

"Miles, if you have any business you need to take care of, I'll be here with Neecy if you need to step out."

"Thanks Monica, I'm good for now."

"Can we go? I still need to make sure the house is ready for tomorrow in case people stop by. We also need to stop by the caterer, and I'm completely exhausted. As they turn to walk out, Neecy stops and looks around. She says out loud, to no one in particular, until tomorrow." As they drive away, Neecy becomes lost in her thoughts. I don't know what tomorrow will bring, but I have to say goodbye to my mother.

Sitting in the front seat on the passenger side, she reaches for Miles free hand hoping to stay grounded, realizing that she needs to feel a human touch for all of this to be real. Miles squeezes her hand to reassure her everything is going to be okay, that she will survive this. At that moment, somehow, she knew she would.

Chapter 20

When The Breath Is Irregular, The Mind Is Unsteady

"Nooo! Noooo, don't!"

"Neecy! Neecy! Miles is screaming Neecy's name but afraid to touch her as Neecy continues to scream, "No." Neecy is shaking, but she is not responding…she keeps screaming. Monica runs into the room to find Neecy squatting behind the door again screaming. Although her eyes are open, she seems to be in some sort of trance and not aware that Monica and Miles are in the room.

"What's wrong with her Monica. Do something!" Monica carefully approaches her, "Neecy, can you hear me?" Monica makes a loud clapping sound with a book she finds nearby. Neecy has a look of confusion on her face as she stares back and forth at Miles and Monica. Her face is wet from the tears, and she is still in a squatting position. "Oh no." she whispers, "please don't tell me it happened again." Miles and Monica are hugging her. Monica asks if she remembers anything that happened. Neecy shakes her head no. All she remembers going to bed and her and Miles discussing the memorial service as she drifted off to sleep.

"Yeah, after I made sure she was asleep, I fell asleep and woke up to find her squatted over in the corner screaming and crying."

"Monica, what's happening? Am I losing my mind or just going crazy?"

"Neither, ride or die. I think the past few days are triggering some memories that you have consciously forgotten."

"Whatever memories you have blocked is your mind's way of protecting you from something that is obviously very painful, it's our body's natural defense mechanism. But now those defenses are breaking down and the memories are starting to manifest, however, they haven't completely emerged from your subconscious to your conscious yet. Basically, because you've blocked the memories, you have never dealt with them. However, it doesn't mean you can't recover memories years or even decades after the event. It often happens spontaneously, and anything can trigger it…a particular smell, taste, or something else related to the suppressed memory. It can come out in therapy as well."

"So, you are telling me I have some demons in my closet that I haven't dealt with?"

"Yes." says Monica. "That's the short version. I'm concerned because we don't know what your memories are, so we don't know what exactly is triggering the memories. So, we don't know how you will respond or what impact it will have on your health when you regain your full memory of what you are blocking."

"You mean my mental health? Are you worried about me going crazy, or that I'm already crazy?"

"Honestly Neecy, I'm concerned about the mental *and* physical impact this can have and is having on you. And no, I don't think you are going crazy."

"Miles looks worried, what now Monica?"

"I recommend that we try to get through the night. Let's try and get some rest and revisit this once the memorial service is over. Neecy, do you want to try and get some rest, or do you want to stay up for a while?"

"I'm exhausted, but I'm afraid to close my eyes. What if this happens again?"

"I think you should try to go back to sleep, if it happens again we will deal with it."

Miles chimes in, "I'm going to be right here, holding you."

"Thank you, Miles."

"I'm in the next room if you guys need me." Monica says as she turns to leave. Neecy hesitantly crawls back into bed. Miles notices her hesitation. "Come on sweetheart, as he stretches out his arms, I'm going to hold you the rest of the night. It's a dream. I won't let any harm come to you. Anyone trying to hurt you will have to go through me first." Neecy settles into Miles' arms and rests her head against his chest. The sound of his heartbeat gently rocks her to sleep.

Chapter 21

Breathe, It's Only A Bad Day If You're Not

"Hello sunshine! God has blessed us with another day!" Patty sings as she enters Angela's room. "I heard you turn on the TV and go to the bathroom, so I knew you were awake. Are you feeling better?"

"A lot better, but I am starving, can we order breakfast?"

"It may be a little late for breakfast, but we can get lunch."

"Lunch, what time is it?"

"It's 1:30 in the afternoon."

"You mean I have been sleeping since yesterday evening?"

"Yes, and I watched over you all night. What do you want to eat?

"Anything is fine Mama...I just need to eat."

"Mama, what about Detective Sherman?"

"He called this morning and I told him I would call him once you were awake to let him know if you were up to continuing the interview."

"Miles also called. He wanted to know how you were doing and if you were up to seeing Neecy. I told him the same, I would call once you were awake."

"Okay, can I eat before I make any decisions about how I feel?"

"No problem, actually the fact that you have your appetite back is a good thing. You are on the road to recovery and things returning to normal."

"I don't know if things will ever be 'normal' again or at least not how we defined normal before all of this happened. Our lives have been forever changed, again. I'm not sure I'm even know what normal is anymore. "

"You have a point, but you must agree better days are on the horizon." Angela smiles at Patty and settles back into her pillow.

"I'm going to get you some food sweetie."

"Thank you Mama."

"Mama did you see this?"

"Neecy held that woman's memorial service today. I wish I had known it was today, I would have gone to support her."

"Yes, I thought about it, but I didn't want to wake you. You are still recovering from a major injury. I know and it may have been best anyway. We don't know that she would have wanted us there."

Patty didn't want to tell her that she had called Detective Sherman about attending and he advised against it. It would crush her heart to know she was asked not to attend. "I guess I can't blame Patrice, she has been through a lot the last few days."

Neecy is overwhelmed when she walks into the memorial service. As she looks around, the chapel is filled with familiar faces. Faces from the hospital. Some attending the services she knows, others she has just seen in passing at the hospital. Nurse Nancy walks up and gives her a big hug.

"Dr. Stromm, I am so sorry for your loss. If there is anything I can ever do don't hesitate to let me know."

Neecy thanks Nancy and then jokingly asks, "Did you guys shut down the hospital?"

"No, but we are on a skeleton crew. Most of us will be heading back as soon as the service is over."

"Nancy, I don't know what to say…thank you."

"There is no need to thank us for coming, we are family. In case you didn't know, this outpouring of people being here today shows how much we love and respect you." Neecy can feel the tears stinging her eyes as Miles squeezes her hand.

Neecy lets Miles guide her to her seat because she can't see through the blur of tears. Neecy thinks to herself, I guess this is what the old saying, 'give me my flowers while I'm alive' means. I would have never thought this many people even knew I existed, let alone cared about me. She lays her head on Miles' shoulder and squeezes Monica's hands as they wait for the service to begin.

Monica looks around the room, recognizing most of the people there. She starts to wonder if Angela and her mother are going to show for the service. It's probably best if they don't. After Miles and I discussed it last night, we are not sure how Neecy would react to them being here, especially since she won't even consider Angela may not have been the aggressor in this situation.

Monica thinks, it's funny how grief can cloud someone's thinking and judgment. Neecy used to tell me about the tirades her mother would go on to the point that they had to leave the house for days at a time. She also has told me about her mother's temper (I've seen it a few times myself) how she could go from 0 to 60 in a blink of an eye. But now she won't even consider her mother could have been trying to hurt Angela, that this may have been self-defense. I certainly wouldn't be surprised if it turns out that way.

Miles looks around the room as subtle as he can without alarming Neecy or disturbing her resting her head on his shoulder. He agreed with Monica last night that maybe Angela and her mother shouldn't come to the service. He was glad that Angela's mother asked Sherm to reach out to him to see what he thought about them attending to support Neecy. If they had shown up, this service could have gone wrong real fast. Sherm told him where they were staying, but since he hasn't finished interviewing Angela about what happened, he wants me to hold Neecy off from talking to her if possible. I told him I would do the best I could, but I can't make any promises. When Neecy makes up her mind about something she can be pretty stubborn about changing it.

Sherm hasn't determined if Angela's story is credible. The day in the hospital when he talked to her she said she couldn't remember what happened. He said there were a lot of holes and she couldn't remember details. But now she is telling the story about what happened without missing a beat, which makes him suspicious. He doesn't know if the time in between interviewing her gave her and her mother time to make up a story about what happened.

"Ladies and gentlemen." Miles' thoughts are interrupted by the funeral director. "Can I have your attention please? The service will start in five minutes. We want to give everyone time to make it to their seats." Everyone stands as the service begins. The minister presiding over the services asks everyone to take their seats. Neecy is sitting between Miles and Monica, she takes a deep breath and squeezes their hands. Here we go. she thinks to herself. I never wanted to be here again. I hope I can make it through this.

The people coming up to Neecy to offer their condolences after the service was over is all a blur. At this point, Neecy realizes how exhausted she is, especially since the past week's sleep has been sporadic at best. She thinks to herself, "Today symbolizes the first day of the rest my life without my mother." She takes Miles hand and asks him to take her home.

As they pull into the driveway, Neecy notices all the cars parked on the block. "Are these people here, at my house?" Miles and Monica look at each other and Miles responds yes. "Remember, we invited everyone to stop by after the service. That's why we hired a caterer." Neecy looks at Miles in a bit of disgust, "I know that Miles, it was a rhetorical question. I'm just surprised at the outpouring of support that I am getting from everyone."

"People love and respect you Neecy, and they want to show their support, even if they didn't know your mother."

As they walk in, Neecy is greeted by friends she hasn't seen since college. Leslie walks up to her and hugs her, Neecy can barely breathe. "Leslie?" "Yes, it's me. When I heard, I had to come and support you. When my brother died in that car accident, I don't know how I would have made it through college without you."

By now, some of Neecy' s other friends have gathered around her. "Neecy you are always there for everyone else, let us take care of you for a change." There is a resounding "yeah" from the crowd.

Neecy looks around the room and starts to cry again. All she can do is nod and motion that she wants to sit down. During the evening, she laughs, she cries, she reminisces about college days. Neecy thinks about how lucky she is…no, how blessed she is, to have people who care about her and show up when she needs them most.

As the evening dwindles and the moon starts to peek out of the sky, the crowd starts to dwindle down. When the last of the guests leave and the caterer has cleaned up and been paid, Neecy turns to Miles and Monica. "I'm tired but not ready to go to bed yet. Monica, you look exhausted, why don't you lie down."

"Are you sure?" Miles interrupts, "It's okay Monica, I'm not sleepy yet. I'll stay up with Neecy for a while."

"The two of you act as if I need a babysitter. I'm not fragile."

"We know. We just want to make sure you are okay." says Monica.

"I'm going to be fine. I'm going to get through this, I promise."

"Well in that case, I'm going to take you up on your offer Miles and go to bed." Monica announces. Neecy turns to Miles, "Now what?"

Miles looks at Neecy and can see the exhaustion in her face, but he dares not point it out to her. Miles thinks to himself that Neecy is afraid to go to sleep because of the nightmares and sleepwalking. Suddenly, a big smile comes over Miles' face, and he goes to the stereo. Neecy smiles at Miles as she hears the smooth sound of King Pleasure's voice coming across the speakers singing "Moody's Mood for Love."

*There I go, There I go, there I go, there... I...go... Pretty baby you are the soul that snaps my control...*Miles sings along as he approaches Neecy. "May I have this dance?" Neecy blushes and takes Miles' hand. They slow dance around the living room, taking in the feel of each other's bodies. Softly breathing, but not saying a word, taking in the mood of the song. Neecy thinks about how much she loves Miles, how she always feels so safe in arms. But she quickly reminds herself of his jealousy and his borderline stalking behavior. If they are going to stay together he has got to change some of his behaviors or their relationship won't last.

As the song comes to an end, Neecy looks up at Miles and says thank you. Miles asks, "Thanks for what?"

"For being you, for staying when I told you to go. Thank you for just being here."

Miles smiles and sings another lyric from the song, "You give me a smile and I am wrapped up in your magic….. There…I go... again…"

Neecy and Miles laugh as they embrace. "Miles." Neecy looks up at him, "I think I can sleep now."

Chapter 22

Breath-Taking Experiences Can Be A Breath Of Fresh Air

Neecy wakes with the sun in her eyes, she moves closer to the middle of the bed expecting to feel the warmth of Miles lying next to her. She keeps scooting in, but no Miles. She reaches out to touch him and he's not there. As she rolls over to look, Miles walks in the door. "Hey Sleepyhead, how are you feeling this fine day?"

"I'm good Miles, what is this?"

"I was coming to see if you were awake so you can eat something."

"Thanks, Miles, what time is it?"

"2 pm"

"2 pm in the afternoon?"

"Yes, two in the afternoon."

"Miles why didn't one of you wake me?"

"Wake you for what, you have somewhere you need to be?"

"No, I guess not, but I have slept half of the day away. I want to try and find Angela and her aunt. I still have some things I need to settle with my mother's estate, but I'm not going to be able to focus until I talk to her. I need to know what happened."

"Neecy, I've talked to Sherm and he thinks you should give it a few more days before you talk to Angela. He said although she has been discharged, she is still recuperating. Let's give it a few more days for her to get her strength back."

"I don't know Miles, what if they leave town?"

"Neecy we already discussed this, Angela paid me a pretty hefty fee to find you. I don't think she is going anywhere until she talks to you."

"What about Detective Sherman, can he tell us anything?"

"Mmmm, I don't know. Let me give him a call and see if he can stop by. In the meantime, I'm going to need you to eat."

"I will and I'm going to get dressed especially if we are about to have company."

"Hey Sherm, yeah this is Miles. I told you I wouldn't be able to distract her. Can you stop by? She asked to speak with you. Tell her what you can that may satisfy her for now. Maybe give you a few more days to get more information and make sure everything checks out before they meet."

"Miles, I don't know how much info I can give her, this is an ongoing investigation, you know the drill. I haven't sorted through everything just yet, they're still some holes in Ms. McMichael's story. I have another meeting with her today in about an hour. I will give you a call after I leave there. If she can provide more information, I may feel more comfortable talking to Dr. Stromm about what we know. On second thought, I can stop by around 6. I have some additional questions for Dr. Stromm as well."

"You have questions for Neecy?"

"Yeah, just some basic background questions."

"Ok Sherm, see you at 6. I'll let Neecy know you are going to stop by." "Neecy, Sherm will be here at 6."

Neecy glances at the clock, "It's almost six now, do you think he will be hungry?"

"I don't know, but I am." Miles says. "I am, too." Monica says standing up, "I will warm some leftovers."

The doorbell rings. Neecy glances at the clock, "He's prompt." she says as she heads for the door.

"Good evening Detective Sherman."

"Good evening Dr. Stromm."

"Please come in." Neecy says as she steps back to make room for Detective Sherman to walk through the door. He's a nice-looking guy Neecy thinks to herself. I wonder if he is married.

"Sherm my man, how are you?" he and Miles shake hands.

"I'm good, how are the two of you doing considering everything that's happened?"

"We are taking it day by day." Neecy manages a smile.

"Sometimes that's all you can do." Detective Sherman looks around thinking to himself, Yep this is how doctors live.

"Dr. Stromm, you have a beautiful home."

"Thank you, Detective."

He pauses at a painting Neecy has hanging in the corridor. "I see you are a fan of Mickalene Thomas?"

"Yes, you know her work?"

"Yes, she was the first to craft an individual portrait of First Lady Michelle Obama and this painting, 'Portrait of Mnonja' was one of my mother's favorites. Thomas's work is an exploration of black female identity, and the way she capitalizes on their natural beauty is powerful."

"Yaaas, her work is powerful."

As he lingers admiring Neecy's collection of artwork, he stops again in front of a large painting that takes up most of the wall in the hallway. "This is a phenomenal work, who is it?"

"It's the 'Aspect of Negro Life in an African Setting' by Aaron Douglas. My mother gave it to me when I graduated from college."

"This is also powerful, the colors and symbolism are mesmerizing."

"Are you an art fan, Detective?"

"I'm an amateur. I grew up in Washington, DC and my mother loved art. She took my brother and I to every art exhibition that came to town, especially if it was an African American exhibition."

"My favorite art exhibition as a kid was William H. Johnson. His folk paintings of faith and family have always stayed with me."

"I have one of his reproductions…let me show you."

"Do you know this one?" Neecy asks pointing to the painting.

"Jitterbug." says Sherm, "it's my favorite."

"Mine too, "However, my favorite artist is Edwin Lester."

"I'm not familiar with his work."

"Oh, I have to show you." Neecy leads Detective Sherman into the den.

Detective Sherman stops in front a picture that takes him into his thoughts as he stands taking in the painting. "This is powerful. Is the artist Edwin Lester?"

"Yes., it is. The painting is a woman's hand holding a spoon. In the spoon is a stack of books, some of the books have titles on the spine, the Bible, Roots. The book on top is open with writing on the page. The page reads American, Slave, Nigger, Colored, Black. The woman is feeding what's in the spoon to a boy who has his mouth open and a tear forming in the corner of his eye."

"Wow this is so realistic, so powerful." Sherm says still in his own thoughts.

"The name of the painting is "Tough Pill To Swallow.""

Detective Sherman looks at Neecy and Miles, "That says it all…"

"Man, let me show you to the living room. Otherwise, Neecy will have you here all night talking about art." As they enter the room, Monica is also walking in. "Good evening Detective Sherman."

"Hello Dr. Armstrong, it's nice to see you again. Likewise, Detective. Are you hungry? I was warming up some food."

"No, Ma'am, I'm on duty."

"No, you're not hungry, or no you don't want to eat because you are on duty?"

Sherm smiles, "I haven't had dinner but I'm on duty and I don't want to impose."

"Non-sense." Neecy says, "if you don't mind leftovers, let's eat and we can talk over dinner."

Detective Sherman smiles, "Well since you twisted my arm, okay."

They go into the dining room where Monica has set the table. "Everything looks great." Sherm says as he takes a seat.

"I wish I could take credit for the meal, but it's leftovers from the catering service yesterday."

"Either way, it all looks good to me Ma'am."

"Let's drop the Ma'am, "you can call me Neecy, and Monica chimes in, "and I'm Monica."

"Very well, Neecy and Monica it is."

As they pass around dishes of food: baked chicken, macaroni and cheese, greens, cornbread muffins, etc., Neecy is the first to break the silence. "So, Detective, what can you tell me about my mother's death?"

"Neecy, can the man get a few bites in before you start grilling him?"

"It's okay Miles, I understand, Neecy is anxious for answers. I will answer what I can, but since it's an ongoing investigation, there may be some information I can't share."

"I understand, Detective, can you tell me what happened? How did my mother die?"

"Ms. McMichael said she went to see your mother at her home to discuss your father. As the conversation continued, the next thing she knew your mother was coming at her with a knife. Your mother murmuring something about her being crazy and how easy it will be to convince the police that Ms. McMichael attacked her. They struggle over the knife and suddenly, Ms. McMichael felt a sharp pain and says that your mother tried to stab her again but somehow, she was able to kick her. Your mother fell back against the stove. She remembers seeing flames and the next thing she knew she woke up in the hospital."

"Did she say what business she had with my father and what her and my mother discussed?"

"No, her memory of events is still foggy and she hasn't fully recovered from her injuries."

"Do you think she is telling the truth?"

"Only time will tell. I still haven't finished interviewing her. She got weak while talking to me the other day so I stopped the interview. I told her we could continue tomorrow if she felt up to it."

Neecy starts to become upset. "If she feels up to it? She is obviously lying. What does she mean she can't remember?"

"Ma'am, I don't know if she is being truthful or not. It's too soon to tell, and we don't want to jump to conclusions."

"How convenient for her to forget certain details. You're a detective, you can't tell that she is lying?"

"Ma'am her not being able to remember details so soon after everything happened is not uncommon."

"With victims of a crime, they often have lapses in memory right after the incident but as time goes on and with rest, they can recall information."

"Oh bull." says Neecy getting angry, she's trying to avoid going to jail."

"Not necessarily Neecy." Monica interrupts. "When anyone, not just victims of a crime, experiences significant trauma, lapse in memory is not uncommon. There have been many studies that show the effects trauma has on the brain. Survivors' immediate reactions in the aftermath of trauma can be very complicated. Their reactions are affected by their own experiences, support network, healing, as well as their coping and life skills."

"Specifically, the memory can be impacted. The person may not be able to tell their story in a linear pattern. When this happens, the assumption is that they are making things up, lying or conveniently omitting parts of the story, when in actuality their memory has been fragmented."

"So, you are saying because of the trauma she's not lying, she just forgot?"

"No Neecy, people do lie, manipulate, recant and change their minds. Come on, you're a doctor, you know how the body works."

Chapter 23

The Mind, The Body, And Breath, They Are All Connected

Detective Sherman looks around the table.

"Dr. Armstrong, Monica. Because I've been doing this for so long, through experience I know that victims often gain their memory back over time, but I have never understood how that all works. Can you tell me more about how the brain works?"

Monica stops eating, she loves her work and any opportunity to talk about trauma and how it impacts our body.

"In my field we refer to it as the stress response. When trauma occurs the amygdala, hippocampus, and prefrontal cortex are affected. The prefrontal cortex (located in the front, outer most layer of your brain) contributes two important elements of recall: Your left frontal lobe stores memories of individual events, your right frontal lobe extracts a theme or main point from a series of events. When trauma occurs, the pre-frontal cortex ability is reduced."

Sherm looks interested, "What do you mean it's reduced?"

"When someone experiences trauma, their prefrontal cortex shuts down and the amygdala takes over. Your amygdala is an almond-shaped mass located deep in your inner brain. It is responsible for emotions and actions, it's the instinctual part of the brain, and it regulates our need for survival. When it detects threats to your survival it:

- Increases your arousal and autonomic responses associated with fear
- Activates the release of stress hormones
- Engages your emotional response
- Decides what memories are stored and where they should be placed
- Applies feeling, tone and emotional charge to memory

"What does that have to do with a victim telling their story? It seems to me that they should be able to remember everything that happened if all of that is taking place."

"It actually has the opposite effect Detective. After trauma a few things can occur:

- Because the amygdala overrides the prefrontal cortex the ability to stop inappropriate reactions or refocus your attention is reduced or non-existent.

- Because of potential decrease in blood flow, you can experience a decreased ability for language, memory, and other functions of the left side of your brain.

- You can also experience increased sadness, anger, anxiety, etc. due to an increase in blood flow to your right prefrontal lobe.

Fear induced by trauma makes a deep imprint on your amygdala and causes it to be oversensitive, which in turn makes it detect threats everywhere, real or perceived. Individuals become hypervigilant to danger even when the danger isn't real."

"Like what happens with people that have PTSD?"

"Yes Detective, exactly. In some PTSD cases, the amygdala has been shown to enlarge through excessive use or complex trauma."

"Can a person recover from PTSD?"

"In some instances, if allowed to heal the damage can change and even reverse the effects."

Sherm looks perplexed, "I'm still not sure I understand how the memory is fragmented."

"Let me explain further. So, the hippocampus is responsible for the formation, organization, storage, and retrieval of memories. It converts short-term memory to long-term memory and sends your memories to the appropriate part of your brain for storage. Trauma blocks the hippocampus from transforming the memories. It stops the memories from being properly integrated. In some cases when the hippocampus' function is suppressed, it has been shown to shrink."

"It shrinks?" Sherm says pondering on what Monica has just explained.

"Yes, it can shrink, but again, resting, allowing healing to take place can reverse the damage. Not always, but if rest can occur, there is a better chance of the brain integrating the memories and repairing any damage that has been done."

"So, it's like having a wound." Sherm begins to get it. If you allow it to heal, there may be a scar but it won't have a long-term effect on functioning of that part of the body. But if your wounded and what may have been just a scar can turn into gangrene if it's not treated properly from the beginning?"

Monica smiles, "Yes that's one way of putting it. Trauma is a wound that happens to the brain. Sometimes it will heal completely and sometimes it won't. There are times that therapy is necessary to assist with healing." Monica glances at Neecy. "It's similar to having a physical injury that you have to go to physical therapy to regain full use of the part of the body that was injured."

"This is fascinating, but I still don't understand why I can have two victims experience the same crime but they react differently."

"Because trauma is subjective. The four of us can be exposed to the same traumatic event and it will impact us differently. Our responses to the same exposer can be vastly different and our behavior reaction can manifest in different ways. For those that have complex trauma, it becomes even more complicated in how the person will respond and what behaviors you will see manifest."

Miles rubs his chin as if in deep thought and asks, "I've heard you say that before. What do you mean by trauma is subjective?"

Monica pauses, "Let me give you an example. One of the biggest mistakes we have seen is with rape victims. The expectation is that they should react in a certain way after a sexual assault occurs. If they are not crying and hysterical immediately after a sexual assault, the assumption is that they are lying."

"Yes." Detective Sherman says, "I've seen that happen when I used to investigate sex crimes. A victim comes in to report a rape. If they are calm and telling their story without any emotion, they get dismissed as not telling the truth for reasons unknown or that they had regret sex."

"Exactly Detective, another response to a traumatic event is what we call toxic immobility. in other words, the 'deer in the headlights' response. For some, when they are exposed to a traumatic event they freeze. This has often happened with rape victims especially if they have experienced more than one assault." Sherm looks perplexed again, "What do you mean more than one assault, do you mean if they are ganged raped?"

159

"Not necessarily, but it can happen in that instance as well. Children of abuse and especially children that have been molested is an example that I like to use. A child that has been molested can experience toxic immobility long into adulthood if they are confronted with a similar experience. Unfortunately, they are blamed and often retraumatized because they didn't scream for help, didn't run, or a term I've heard too often, 'they just laid there' so they must have wanted it to happen."

Sherm leans forward, toward Monica, excited about the conversation. "So, tell me about the different responses, why would the four of us respond differently if exposed to the same situation?" Monica smiles at his excitement.

She continues, "Studies have shown that when we are exposed to danger and the brain does what I just explained, there is also a hormonal chemical release that happens. That chemical release of hormones varies from person to person. It would be the same as trying to explain why some get cancer and others don't. There are so many factors that come into play and the variation of the release of hormones. I've heard it referred to as a hormonal cocktail. When the brain signals that danger is occurring, our bodies releases a flood of hormones to help you respond to the perceived or real danger.

"As these hormones surge through the bloodstream, it causes the heart to beat faster and primes the body for an emergency. It also signals various parts of the brain to supercharge the intense emotional memory of the traumatic event you are experiencing. The National Institute of Justice generated a study on Sexual Assault by Dr. R. Campbell. The study revealed the main chemicals that are released by the adrenals during a traumatic event. These are the hormones that course through the body to help with the "fight" response, if the body was going to be fighting back against the traumatic event that's happening to it."

"The hormones might also be useful if the response is to "flee" the situation, try to run away to try to get away from the threatening situation. These hormones are helpful for the fight-or-flight response. In conjunction with that, we have cortisol. Cortisol levels are going to affect the amount of energy that the body has to fight back or to try to flee the situation."

"Because traumatic events often involve physical pain in addition to emotional pain, two other hormones might be released by the adrenals, opiates the natural morphine in our body to try to compensate for the physical and emotional pain. And in conjunction with the morphine is oxytocin. The oxytocin is released to try to increase positive feelings. In essence, the body is trying to make sure that it is managing the physical pain during a traumatic event."

"That's fascinating. It's too bad that all of my law enforcement counterparts don't have this information. Wait until I get back to the station and start kicking this knowledge to everyone. Thanks Dr.

Armstrong for the information, this will gain a lot traction for victims we encounter."

"No problem, and if you ever want a presentation to your law enforcement or judicial partners, give me a yell. I think it is so important for the judicial system to understand what's happening in the body. It could change the way the judicial system conducts investigations and prosecute cases for the better of the victim."

Sherm and Miles nod their heads in agreement.

Chapter 24

All In The Same Breath

Monica turns to Neecy, "So Neecy all that I am saying is that we need to give her time to see if she remembers anything else or if she can provide more detail about what happened. Her story may change, or as Detective Sherman investigates the case, he may find out that she is lying about what happened. We just can't jump to conclusions because of the behavior being displayed so early after a major traumatic event."

"I know Monica and thanks for reminding me. It's just that it's my mother and I want answers. I need to understand what happened."

"I know, Dr. Stromm." says Sherm, "and I'm going to do everything within my power to get to the truth."

"Thank you Detective, I know you are doing everything you can." Another question, when do you think I can talk to her? Can you give me her contact information?"

"I don't know Ma'am, but I can tell you that she and her mother are anxious to speak with you. I will reach out to them to find out if it's okay to give you their contact information."

"Thank you, you also have my permission to give them my contact information."

"Detective, how is the food?" Monica says to try and break up some of the tension in the room.

"It's great. I haven't had a home-cooked meal in a while. As a bachelor, your first order of business isn't to cook."

"You're a bachelor, Detective?" Neecy asks as she kicks Monica under the table.

Monica catches Sherm staring and begins to blush as she flashes him one of her winning smiles.

"Yes, I'm single, I haven't found 'the one'."

"Mmmm." Neecy thinks to herself, I'm going to have to see what I can do about that.

Sherm catches himself staring at Monica and quickly reminds himself not to stare at her but can't seem to help himself. Sherm thinks to himself how he could easily get lost in Monica's big beautiful eyes, her perfect smile and her caramel colored skin.

"Would you like dessert or coffee Detective?" Neecy asks while winking at Monica?

"No thank you, Ma'am." Neecy interrupts, "it's Neecy." Sherm smiles, "No thank you, Neecy. I better get going, I have an early morning. Thank you again for dinner."

"Hey man, thanks for coming over." "I will walk you to the door. As Sherm and Miles stand up from the table, Neecy and Monica in unison, "Goodbye Detective."

"Hey Sherm, has Angela said anything else about the letter?"

"Not yet, I'm going to ask more about the contents of the letter when I meet with her again. Her mother showed up, so I didn't want to get into details. You know how that can go if there are things the victim may not want a loved one to know. I talked to her in her hotel room. I'm going to ask her if she will come to the station for the next interview so that I can speak to her alone."

"Thanks again, I appreciate you keeping me in the loop."

"No problem, until we know the whole story and if Angela's story checks out we need to keep Neecy safe. I wouldn't have had as much info that I have if you hadn't filled in some of the blanks. I better get going."

"Ok man, later."

Miles closes and locks the door and takes a deep breath. He thinks to himself, I hope this is over soon so that we can get to the business of us. I know Neecy feels like I betrayed her, hopefully when the truth comes out she will understand why I handled this situation the way I did. What I need her to know is that I never meant to fall for her, it happened before I even realized what was happening. When I realized I was violating one of my own rules, not to get personal with someone I'm investigating, I should have come clean then and recused myself from the case. But, it's too late to focus on woulda, coulda, shoulda's. I'm going to have to deal with the aftermath of my decisions good or bad. Miles, hears Neecy calling his name. "Miles, do you want dessert or coffee?" "Coming babe, I'll have some coffee."

Later that evening Neecy is sitting in bed reading some Yoga literature Monica gave her. As Miles crawls into bed, he glances at the title. "What are you reading?" "Oh, this is some yoga literature Monica gave me about breathing. Listen to this. Experts stress that proper breathing is a science and an art, it's something we have to learn."

Miles looks confused, "We have to learn to breathe, isn't that something we do naturally."

"Yes and no, for example, when someone is in physical distress we tell them to take deep breaths, it helps to slow the heart rate and calm the nerves. Breathing can also be effective when you are stressed. When you feel the stress in your shoulders, neck and back, deep breathing exercises can help to release the stress and release the tension created by the stress."

"Interesting." Miles says as he processes the information. "The literature goes on to say that better breathing keeps us healthy. Breathing can calm us, it can give us more energy, and the deeper we breathe, the better we feel. What most don't realize is that the mind, body, and breath are intimately connected and influence each other. Our breathing influences our thoughts, and our thoughts and physiology can be influenced by our breath."

"That's fascinating, so the way we breathe is connected to our health."

"Yes, and our health is connected to our breathing."

"Can I read that when you are finished?"

"Of course, Miles."

"I'm going to sleep do you need anything before I crash?"

"No, I'm going to read some more, I'm not sleepy." Neecy begins to think about what Monica said at dinner. Have I experienced some significant trauma? Is that why I can't remember my life at six years old, why details prior to six are fuzzy? Are my nightmares and sleepwalking because of some forgotten trauma? Do Angela and her mother hold the key to my memories? And most confusing, what does my mother have to do with all of this?

Neecy continues to think to herself, I'm curious but at the same time afraid to find out. What if I have experienced something so traumatic I can't handle it. After all, if there's any truth to it, that's why I blocked the memory in the first place. This is all so overwhelming, I guess my only option is one day at a time. I have to let this unfold in the manner its intended to reveal itself and pray that I don't lose my mind in the process.

Chapter 25

Make Every Breath Count

Neecy wakes up the next morning, and the house is unusually quiet. She walks through the house calling out for Miles and Monica, but no one answers. As she is turning to leave the kitchen, she notices the note. Neecy, I didn't want to wake you. I had to go into the office to take care of some things. Miles left this morning, he said he had to follow up on a lead for a case he is working. I will be back around 4.

Miles left this morning? What time is it? Oh My God! It's 3 in the afternoon! I can't believe I have slept the day away. Neecy thinks to herself, Angela may not be ready to talk, but that doesn't mean I can't research who she is. Neecy jumps on her laptop and googles Angela McMichael. Several Angela's come up in the search. Neecy clicks on a picture of Angela McMichael. As Angela's information comes up, Neecy is still blown away by how much they look alike. The picture includes an article written about Angela.

Alright, Ms. McMichael who are you? Wow, she has an impressive portfolio. She is a prominent attorney in the North Carolina area. Her law firm has made millions by representing victims of crime in lawsuits and defending victims who have been accused of crimes. Attorney Angela McMichael's leads her law firm in ensuring victims not only know their rights, but she also ensures victims' rights are protected. Her practice includes representation for victims of:

- Child Sexual Abuse
- Rape/sexual assault
- Sexual Harassment
- Domestic Violence
- Wrongful Death
- Assault and battery

She has defended clients in successful third-party lawsuits against security companies, schools, hospitals, nursing homes, employers, hotels, apartment complexes, universities, day care centers and churches. "I bet she has some interesting stories about lawsuits against the church Neecy says out loud but to no one in particular."

"Who are you talking to?" Neecy is startled, she didn't hear anyone come in. "Oh Monica, it's you, I thought you weren't going to be back until 4?"
"It's 4:15 Neecy."

"OMG! I didn't realize it was getting so late."

"Neecy, what are you reading?"

"I decided to google Ms. Angela McMichael's."

"Oh, what did you find out?"

"Here read for yourself." Neecy says standing up

169

and handing Monica her laptop. "I need to take a shower, we can talk after I get dressed." Neecy turns on the shower and steps in as the water is getting hot. I don't know what to think at this point. How much does Miles know about this Angela? What is it that Detective Sherman can't tell me? I know he wasn't telling me everything he knows about this case. The biggest question is why the secrets and why are they keeping them from me?

Neecy lets the water run on her face, down the back of her neck and shoulders. As the water is running it dawns on her, "If Miles was investigating her, he definitely knows more about this entire situation than what he is telling." She asks herself if she is sleeping with the enemy. Don't be silly Neecy, if Miles was here to hurt you he has had plenty of opportunity in the past year to hurt you. But what is he hiding? Does Monica know any of this? She was suddenly very supportive of Miles when this all started.

Somebody is going to tell me something. Neecy hurries to get dressed and finds Monica in the den. "Ok Monica, are you ready to tell me what's going on? Monica looks up at Neecy with a confused look. I know you Monica. You couldn't stand Miles. Especially after we found out that Miles has been lying about who he is. Any other time you would have started the campaign for me to give him his walking papers, but instead, you keep encouraging me to hear him out. Now, all of sudden you guys have become buddies. I want to know and I want to know now, what's going on?"

Monica sighs and tells Neecy to sit down. "I do know more than what I was telling you Neecy. I don't know the whole story, but that day in the hospital, when we thought it was you that was brought into the emergency room, Miles confessed to me who he was and why he has been deceptive."

"And you kept that from me?"

"For now, I had every intention of telling you what I knew after we got through your mother's memorial service and you had a few days to grieve."

"Ok, I've had a few days, start talking."

"Neecy, don't blame Monica." Neecy and Monica turn to see Miles standing in the doorway. "This is all on me. I swore Monica to secrecy and wouldn't tell her anything about Angela or why I was trying to find you until she gave me her word she wouldn't say anything before it was time."

"Once Miles told me what he knew about why Angela was looking for you, I agreed not to say anything for now because I wasn't sure how you would handle everything at one time."

"What is everything? And I wish everyone would quit treating me as if I'm some fragile china doll that has to be handled with care."

"Neecy, we haven't meant any disrespect toward you, we just wanted to make sure you were ok."

"What's so terrible that you have to make decisions about me without me having a say in the decision. The two of you have made decisions for me, that will impact me, and I don't get a say in the decision? This is the ultimate disrespect in minimizing my ability to speak for myself. When was I going to have a say about who I let in my life and when?"

"Neecy, Angela asked Sherm if he would relay the message for you to call her. Here is her phone number."

"I'm surprised you didn't try to call and talk to her on my behalf without me knowing, or did you and Monica decide you would do that for me?"

"Neecy we were only trying to look out for you."

"Yeah, Monica, I get that, but when was I going to have a say in what I do?"

Miles touches Neecy's arm, "you can have a say now Neecy. You can call Angela and arrange to meet her."

"The two of you are not going to drive me crazy. I'm putting both of you on pause. I left my phone in the bedroom. I'm going to call her and arrange to meet so we can talk. Maybe I will finally be able to get to the bottom of all this."

Neecy walks out of the room. Miles and Monica look at each other.

"Whoa, she is putting us on pause…. I've never heard her use that phrase."

"I have and it's not good. In fact, in all the years I've known her I've only heard her use that phrase with someone twice. It means she is pissed. There is nothing you or I can say or do right now to get back in her good graces. A good sign is that she didn't tell us she was pissed off to the highest of pisstivity."

Miles looks perplexed, "to the highest of pisstivity?"

"Yeah, that's a word she made up the first time I heard her use the phrase that she was putting someone on pause, it was to emphasize how upset she was."

"Miles ask, so what do we do?"

Monica shakes her head, 'nothing, our best bet right now is to wait it out, give her time to cool down. Maybe we will be able to talk about this later, much later."

Neecy comes back in the room. "I am meeting Angela and her mother at 7 pm at her hotel. She is still in recovery but saw her doctor today, they removed the stitches and he said the wound is healing nicely. But I still don't want her trying to get dressed and take a car ride over here or to meet somewhere."

"Neecy, I know you are upset with us right now, but I would like to go with you if you let me. However, if you want to go alone I will respect your decision."

"The same for me ride or die, I would like to go, but will respect your wishes either way."

"Of course, I want the two of you to go with me. I still need the support and I don't think I should meet with them by myself. But know that this does not set us straight, we can deal with all of this later. I can only deal with one thing at a time. Right now this takes priority over anything the two of you have done, agreed? Agreed, Miles and Monica respond at the same time."

The car ride to the hotel was in silence, only the music on the radio prevented the ride from dead silence. Miles is driving and Monica is sitting in the front seat, Neecy is in the backseat. When they walked out to the car Neecy told Monica, "Uh Uh, since you and Miles have become such good buddies you sit in the front so that I can keep my 'good eye' on both of you." Miles has the radio on the Oldies but Goodies radio station.

When the song by the Three Degrees comes on, I Didn't Know... The Three Degrees is singing I didn't know, oooh, you were gonna be my baby. I didn't know loving you would drive me crazy…. Miles smiles thinking this is our song… Neecy leans closer to the front and in almost a whisper while smiling, "Miles…" "Yeah, baby, do you want me to turn this up?" "No, I want you to turn it off, it's getting on my nerves." Miles smile quickly fades. Monica keeps her head and eyes straight to the front. The remainder of the ride is in dead silence.

When they finally arrive at the hotel, Miles gives the valet his keys. Neecy has already headed toward the door, not waiting for Miles or Monica.

Miles looks at Monica and whispers "what do I do?"

"I told you nothing, just give her some time. We better catch up." They catch up with Neecy at the elevator.

Neecy is starting to feel some anxiety, so she starts taking some deep breaths. Monica notices her breathing has changed. "Neecy are you ok?"

"I'm a little nervous, I just got this feeling in the pit of my stomach that what I'm about to hear is going to change my life forever. I just can't tell if the change is going to be a good change or a not so good change."

Miles starts to grab Neecy's hand, but then has second thoughts. "We are here for you Neecy, whatever you need." "I know Miles", she gives him a half smile and reaches out her hand.

They exit the elevator holding hands. Monica has her arm entwined with Neecy's. Neecy must really be nervous Miles thinks to himself, her palms are sweaty.

I'm too mad at them to tell them how much I appreciate them being here right now. I don't think I would have been able to do this by myself.

Chapter 26

When One Breath Isn't Enough, Take Two

Neecy rings the doorbell of the suite. Here we go she says under her breath. A few seconds later Patty answers the door and invites them in. After cordial greetings Neecy tells Patty, "I hope it's ok that I brought my boyfriend and best friend."

"Yes, of course. PattyCake, I mean Angela told me you were bringing them. Please come in and have a seat, I'll go and get Angela."

The three of them walk into the living space of the suite taking it all in to include the breath-taking view of the mountains. Miles thinks to himself, wow I knew she was well off, but this, this suite is easily five grand a night and that's only because we are in Colorado. I can't imagine what it would be if we were in LA or DC. Miles thoughts are interrupted by Neecy, "isn't' this view breathtaking?"

"Yeah, Monica says starring out the window, who can't recover in this place."

As Angela walks into the room with Patty holding her arm, Miles rushes over to assist her to the lounge chair in the room. As Angela eases into the lounge chair, "thank you for coming Neecy, I know this has all been suspenseful for you."

"Thank you for reaching out, it has been, and I

know you are still recovering so I will try not to exhaust you."

"No worries, as I told you on the phone, I'm as anxious for us to talk as you are."

"But you first, what questions can I answer for you?"

"I think the obvious question is why you went to see my mother and what happened between the two of you that it resulted in my mother's death."

Angela looks at Patty, takes a deep breath and begins to tell Neecy why she was looking for her. When she gets to the part about the letter, Neecy stops her. "What letter?" "You received a letter from my father?" "Yes, I received a letter from our father."

"What do you mean our father? I don't have any siblings."

"Yes, Neecy you do, I'm your sister. In fact, we are twins."

"Liar!" Neecy yells liar so loud it startles everyone in the room.

Monica rushes over and sits next to Neecy. "Neecy sweetie are you Ok? Do you want her to go on?"

Neecy glares at Angela and then nods her head,

"yes go on. I can't wait to hear this." Angela looks at Patty and asks her if she can get the letter from her briefcase.

Miles is sitting next to Neecy with his arm around her waist. Patty returns with the letter and hands it to Angela. Angela glances at the letter and hands it to Neecy. "Do you recognize the handwriting?" Neecy takes the letter. As soon as she sees the handwriting, her hands begin to tremble to the point that she drops the letter.

"How did you get a letter with my father's handwriting?"

"Neecy, I have no reason to lie, this is a letter from our father that was mailed to me a little over a year ago. That's what started this whole sequence of events, I hired Miles to look for you. I just never imagined it would happen like this."

"Feel free to take the time to read the letter if you need more proof. I have nothing but time." Neecy picks the letter up off the floor and hands it back to Angela. "I can't read it right now, what does the letter say?" Angela looks around the room, Patty moves closer to her as they both begin to feel the tears stinging their eyes. "Neecy, Angela begins, do you remember what happened when we were six?" Neecy now looks confused, "what does us being six have to do with this letter?"

"Do you remember anything about us, about what

happened when we were six?" Neecy starts to ask the question again, but Monica interrupts. "Neecy sweetie, you have been searching for answers, it's time. Only being transparent and honest is going to yield the answers you have been looking for." Neecy nods her head and looks at Angela. "No, I can't remember anything about that time, that age is a total blank to me as if I didn't exist during that time. I can only remember bits and pieces of my life prior to six, it's all fuzzy."

"It may be because that's when Patrice Stanford ceased to exist and Shanice Stromm was born." Neecy half laughs and says what are you talking about? Patty is now praying under her breath, "sweet Jesus, she really doesn't remember. How can this be? Sweet Jesus, help us." Angela continues, "It was also when Patricia Stanford ceased to exist, and Angela McMichael's was born."

"You're not making any sense right now." Neecy says in an irritated voice. "Neecy, we are twins. Our mother use to always dress us alike. Our favorite outfit was a striped red shirt and some denim shorts with white sneakers. In the summertime mama had to wash those outfits two or three times a week because that's all we ever wanted to wear."

Neecy looks at Angela, "how do you know about my dream?"

Now Angela looks confused, "Your dream, what dream?"

"I often have a dream of me as a little girl playing with a girl that looks like me. We are dressed alike and we... are... identical." Neecy voice traces off as she realizes her dream may have been a memory of her playing with Angela. Neecy turns to Monica, "Monica is this possible? Is it possible that I was dreaming about playing with Angela, that this wasn't a symbolic dream, but instead a memory?"

"It's very possible Neecy, in fact, it sounds like its real." Monica turns to Angela, Angela can you tell us more about your childhood with Neecy before you turned six?"

"Yes, those were happy times. We lived in this big house with our parents. Our mother was about our complexion and beautiful. I remember her always daunting over us. She used to tell us how special we were, how beautiful we were and that we were going to take the world by storm when we were older. She always told us that we were twins because when God created the first one, he was so pleased with his work that he had to repeat it."

Angela smiles as she reminisces about their mother. "I was a mama's girl, always hanging out in the kitchen with her, cooking, baking, etc. Neecy you were a daddy's girl. Whenever you saw daddy, you saw Neecy, she went everywhere with him."

There were not a lot of kids on the block our age so most of the time it was just Neecy and I playing together. We were closer than close and always looked out for each other."

"If all of this is true, then why don't I remember any of it?"

Monica looks at Neecy, "Neecy I think it's because of the trauma you were exposed to when you were six." Neecy sighs, "What trauma?"

Angela looks at Patty. Patty shifts her weight, takes a deep breath and begins to explain. "Neecy, when you were six there was a house fire. Until that letter arrived, we thought you and your father had died in the fire along with your mother. All these years we thought you were dead. If we had known you were alive we would not have stopped looking for you until we found you."

"Died with my mother? What are you people talking about? My mother raised me. I just buried my mother because of you." Neecy is glaring at Angela. Miles is now gently squeezing Neecy's hand and whispers in her ear, "Baby let them finish." Patty has tears streaming down her face, shakes her head and says, "No Neecy, your mother died in a house fire when you were six."

"How can that be true? What about my father?
"You said you thought both of us were dead. Now I guess you're going to tell me my father wasn't my father?"

Patty is now looking empathetic toward Neecy.

"No Neecy, you were raised by your father, the letter, the handwriting, it's his handwriting."

"How do you know it was his handwriting?"

"Because he was my baby brother." Neecy is now half laughing, "so now you're telling me you are my aunt. Well how are you my aunt and Angela's mother, but we are twin sisters?" Patty wipes her tears and clears and takes a deep breath. "Your father's real name was Dale, Dale Stanton. We grew up together in North Carolina. We use to be thicker than thieves and I adored your mother."

"My mother Alice?" Patty shakes her head, "no Neecy, your birth mother."

"When you guys were five, your birth mother and my brother briefly separated. During that time Dale met Alice and they had an affair. Soon after they became involved, Dale realized that he really loved your mother and couldn't bear the thought of the two of you growing up without him, he didn't want to be a part-time father. So, he ended the affair with Alice and moved back home with the two of you and your mother. Angela doesn't remember any of this, probably because you were too young and their separation was brief (about six months). He told me several times, the worst mistake he ever made was leaving his family."

"So if this is true how did he end up with my mother Alice? Angela chimes in, "all these years we didn't know he was with Alice until the letter showed up."

"Neecy sounding frustrated asks, "what is it with this letter, do I need to read it?" You can read it now if you would like." Angela says holding out the letter to Neecy. Neecy looks at the letter, hesitating even to hold it, this is it, she says to herself. If I read the contents of this letter, it will forever change the course of my life. "I'm not ready to read the letter, go on with your story." Angela nods and takes a deep breath before continuing.

"When the letter arrived, it starts off with if you are reading this I'm already dead. Our father says in the letter that he is writing it in his hand writing so that we would know it came from him. I didn't know our daddy's handwriting being that I was so young when he left. I took the letter to Aunt Patty. She immediately recognized his handwriting."

"The letter explained that he didn't die in the house fire. He explains in the letter that he has been in hiding, or should I say hiding in plain sight with you and Alice."

"But why? Why did they need to hide out?"

Neecy is sitting between Miles and Monica, they glance at each other because they have already figured out where this story is going. Monica thinks to herself, I hope Neecy can handle what she is about to hear. Monica is contemplating if she should stop them, they still don't know what Neecy was exposed to or saw, or how deep the trauma goes. Since she doesn't have those answers, she doesn't know how this will impact Neecy. It could force her into a deeper level of denial or worse.

Monica interrupts Angela, "I'm sorry to interrupt, but can we take a break I need to talk to Neecy." "Now Monica? Are you serious? Right now?"

"Baby, maybe you should hear Monica out before they continue."

"There you two go, trying to make decisions for me. No, I want to continue." Monica turns toward Neecy. "Neecy, you have blocked any memory of what you have heard thus far, I'm concerned that what you may hear next can do more damage."

"Angela and Patty, please forgive my friend and boyfriend, they seem to think I can't handle myself. And my friend the psychologist here thinks she knows what best for my mental health. Neecy that's not what I'm saying at all." Patty interrupts, "You are a psychologist?" "Yes, ma'am, I specialize in trauma."

"Well look at how God works." Patty chuckles to herself, "your best friend is a trauma specialist."

"Neecy, maybe you should listen to your friend. I had to take Angela to a trauma specialist after everything happened. She did wonders for Angela's wellbeing." "Wonders" Angela says, "she worked

185

miracles. The nightmares stopped and I was able to move through the grief of losing my family."

Chapter 27

With Bated Breath

"I agree with Monica and Mama, maybe we are moving too fast. I know firsthand the havoc trauma can wreak on your mental health, which then can affect your physical health." Monica pleads with Neecy. "Neecy, everyone in this room not only cares to about you, we also love you and care about your wellbeing." "Yeah Neecy, we aren't going anywhere, I'm prepared to stay in Colorado for as long as it takes." Patty chimes in, "That's right Suga Plum...that's what I used to call you, now that we have found you, we aren't going anywhere."

"Ok, I'm willing to pause, but I'm not leaving here until I hear the whole story." Miles says in a loud voice, "Oh boy, she is digging in, we all better prepare for a long night. Angela, how are you feeling?"

"I'm good, a little hungry, would you guys like to order room service, the hotel restaurant has a leg of lamb meal to die for." Monica frowns, "No lamb for me, what else do they have?"

"I like the steak myself, I've had it almost every night since we checked in" says Patty. "I'll have what she is having." Monica says, Miles chime in "count me in for the steak too. Neecy chuckles, "I have never been able to resist a good leg of lamb." For the first time, she looks over at Angela and smiles.

As they eat at the dining table in the hotel suite, Neecy tells Angela, "You're right this is one of the best legs of lambs I've ever had." "Told you..." As they are finishing their meals, Neecy asks Angela to tell her more about her practice. "It's pretty simple. I defend victims of all types of crime." "How did you come about choosing that particular area of law?" "After the fire I went to live with Mama." Angela smiles and looks over at Patty. "I call her Mama despite her protest because she took me in and raised me as her own.

"After going to live with Mama, a detective showed up at our door one day to tell us they were closing the case because they didn't have any more leads. He also told Mama that I could be in potential danger because they still didn't know exactly what happened the night of the explosion. When Mama tried to press for more information the Detective told her he couldn't tell her any more information."

Patty interjects, "Imagine my frustration when this man, a law enforcer, tells me my baby is in danger, but he can't give me any information. It made no sense to me. I asked for protection and he said because they were closing the case, all he could do is issue me a warning that she could be in danger. Imagine that, issue me a warning as if he were giving me a parking ticket. We were all terrified at that point, not just for Angela but for our family because he left us with no information. He just told me to be careful and left."

"That's all he said?"

"Yes, since he wouldn't tell me why he thought Angela might be in danger, I hired a victim's right attorney. It's amazing what we don't know about our rights. I didn't know at the time victims had rights until I started looking for an attorney that could help me get information from the police. A good friend introduced me to the victims' rights attorney. She got the information from the police that we needed to know how to protect Angela, which by the way was our right to know (I'm sure there was some information the police couldn't release). She also connected us with a Victim Advocate who helped connect us with resources and services we needed.

"The information the police had not given us could have left Angela in danger. The attorney recommended and helped us legally change your sister's name so she would be harder to find in case she was in danger. We chose Angela McMichael.

"The Victim Advocate connected us with the trauma specialist for Angela." "Neecy looks curious, what was your name before you changed it?" "It was Patricia Stanford. We were named after Aunt Patty. My name was Patricia, and your name Neecy was Patrice Stanford."

"What, my name was Patrice?" "Yes Suga Plum, I used to call you Suga Plum and Angela I have always called PattyCake."

189

"My name was Patrice? Who changed my name and why?'

"The letter explained that they changed your name because you were already presumed dead, and they wanted Patrice to stay dead."

"Angela, what kind of danger were you in that your name had to be changed?"

Angela looks at Monica."I'm sorry, I didn't mean to bring it back to the conversation of what has happened." "It's ok, as you get to know Neecy, you will learn that once she has her mind set on something it's hard to avoid giving her answers. It's so ironic because I tell her all the time she should have been a lawyer instead of a doctor." "Amen to that." Miles says out loud. "All of you are talking about me as if I'm not sitting here. Since we are back to the topic at hand can we continue with what's in the letter?"

"Are you sure you are up to it Suga Plum?" "Yes, ma'am I'm sure. Besides. Neecy thinks to herself, if I'm going to let her continue to call me Suga Plum, somebody better make all of this make sense to me. "What about you PattyCake, how are you feeling? You don't want to wear yourself out."

"I'm good Mama, I'm willing to continue if Neecy wants to continue." "There it's settled. I have made up my mind to continue." Neecy says as she leans back in her chair. "I want to know what the letter says."

Patty stands up, "well it's settled, why don't we move back to the living room where everyone can get comfortable while I make some coffee and bring dessert? I picked up a carrot cake from the little bakery down the street and it is delicious." Everyone nods as they get up from the table. Miles helps Angela back to the lounge chair as Patty heads toward the kitchen.

Once Angela is settled in the lounge chair, Neecy props pillows behind her head. "Comfortable?" "Yes, thank you. I'm ready to answer your questions. What we found out was that my mother, our mother was murdered. The police thought that the person that killed the rest of my family may still be after me. Because I didn't have a lot of information to help with the investigation, they were never able to come up with a suspect or a motive. All they were ever able to determine was that one of the neighbors saw a car speeding away just before the house exploded. In the letter Daddy said they changed everyone's last name to Stromm and your first name was Shanice, but they called you Neecy."

"Why did they think my father and I died in the fire?"

"Because his car and our mother's car were still parked in the driveway. Some of the neighbors said they had seen him come home about an hour before the explosion. Because you stuck to daddy like glue and we couldn't find you, they concluded that you also died when the house exploded from the gas leak."

"What started the gas leak? We are not sure, and its information the police wouldn't give us. All they would say is that a gas burner on the stove had been left on. They wouldn't say if it was intentional or not, especially since I told them that Mama had cooked dinner. They said she could have left the burner on by accident. All that I know is there are holes in their investigation. There are things we may never know."

"Wait, you said our mother was murdered?"

"Yes, murdered. The autopsy revealed that our mother was dead before the fire was set because there was no smoke in her lungs. The coroner noted that she had been strangled and stabbed. However, he couldn't determine which killed her."

"She was strangled" Neecy voice trails off.

"OMG! OMG!" Neecy starts screaming. Patty runs into the living room. "OMG! I remember, I remember everything!" Neecy starts crying and then hyperventilating. Monica grabs her hands as the others look on with worry. "Monica, I remember!"

"I remember what happened! I remember every detail. OMG! How could I have forgotten!"

Miles is holding Neecy, "how could you have

forgotten what baby?"

In between sobs Neecy says, "how could I have forgotten that I witnessed my mother's murder?"

Chapter 28

Remember To Breathe

Monica tries to maintain her composure at the shock of the news so that she can stay in the frame of mind to help Neecy. Miles is standing watching Neecy and feels helpless, he wasn't expecting this. Monica gently squeezes Neecy's hand. "Neecy, can you feel me squeezing your hand? If so just nod." Neecy nods. Good Monica says to herself and thinks at least we haven't lost her. Miles steps back so that Monica is standing in front of Neecy. "Neecy, remember the breathing technique I taught you?" Neecy nods her head. "Ok, let's do it together."

"Inhale, 1,2,3, 4, hold 1,2,3,4,5,6,7, exhale blowing out through your mouth, 1,2,3,4,5,6,7,8. Nice, let's do it again." As Monica is helping Neecy, Miles turns and glares at Angela and Patty, "You knew this all along, and you didn't think you should tell me?" Angela is shocked by Miles anger. "Miles, I wasn't intentionally keeping this from you, I wasn't trying to hide anything."

"After I told you I had fallen in love with your sister you didn't think I should have known she witnessed a murder and not just any murder, her own mother's murder!"

"Miles, I'm sorry, I didn't know she actually witnessed what happened. All the letter says is that she suffered some significant trauma and there was no indication that she remembered what happened. I don't know what else to say, I wasn't trying to hide it. I didn't know."

Monica looks back at Miles, "Miles this isn't the time, we need to focus on Neecy."

"You're right Monica, Neecy are you okay?" Neecy is still crying but has calmed down enough to speak.

"Yes, I'll be okay."

"Don't be upset with Angela, none of us are handling this very well. It's not like there is an instruction book on how to handle this type of situation." Neecy looks at Angela. "Is this what was in the letter?" Angela is also crying, "He only said you saw something you shouldn't have seen but there was no indication that you remembered. Neecy I am so sorry. I'm not trying to cause any more confusion than there already is, I just want my sister back."

Neecy walk over to Angela and hugs her. "It's okay, the truth had to come out. I needed to remember if we were ever going to reconnect."

Angela looks at Neecy, "You want to reconnect?"

"Yeah Sis, I just said I remember. I remember that day. Daddy had been at work all day and Mama had baked a chocolate cake for dessert after dinner. We couldn't wait for daddy to get home so we could eat dinner and then have some cake."

"We had played all day together outside in our favorite outfit, the red striped shirt, and denim shorts. We were trying to learn how to Double Dutch like we had seen on TV. Since we didn't have anyone else to turn the rope while one of us jumped, we had tied one end of the rope to handles on the garage." "Yes, Angela says laughing, we kept tripping on the rope because the ends tied to the garage were to close together."

Neecy pauses and starts to cry again. "Neecy are you ok?" "Yes, Monica, I'm fine. I have to do this now. I don't want to take a break or I may never get it out." As everyone is standing around Neecy, she continues. "Daddy came home and we kept waiting for dinner. Instead, Mama called us in the kitchen and gave us each a slice of cake. She seemed upset, but we were kids and happy that we didn't have to wait for dinner before we could have some cake."

"After we finished our cake mama told us she had to run a quick errand, to take our baths. Angela you lost rock, scissors, paper, so you had to take your bath first. I watched TV for a minute waiting for you to finish and decided to look for daddy. I heard his voice in their bedroom. He was arguing with someone, it was a female voice, but it didn't sound like mama. When I walked in daddy was arguing with a woman I had never seen before. He was asking her how she got in their house, in their bedroom. He kept telling her that she needed to leave before his wife got back."

"They were going at each other so intensely they didn't even notice I was in the room. The woman smiled and sat on the bed and said she wasn't going anywhere, she was waiting for Daddy to come home. Daddy was yelling by now and screamed at the woman he was home and she was crazy. About that time, Mama walked in the room, but by that time I had already squatted behind the door so she didn't see me when she walked in the room."

"Mama asked what was going on and asked the lady why she was there. The woman repeated that she was there to take her man home. Mama told her that she has had enough of her foolishness. It was time to give it up, Daddy obviously didn't want to be with her, or he wouldn't have moved back home. Mama emphasized the word home and when she did the woman went crazy. She lunged for mama and grabbed her by the throat. Daddy had to wrestle the woman to the ground to get her to let go of Mama."

"Once she let go of Mama, Mama was sitting on the bed coughing and Daddy turned to Mama to ask if she was ok. That's when the woman really went crazy. She started screaming at Daddy about how dare he ask her if she was ok in front of her. Suddenly, the woman pulled out a knife and lunged at Daddy. Mama jumped in front of Daddy trying to push him out of the way. That's when the woman stabbed Mama."

"I can remember Mama's eyes. They got big as saucers as the pain shot across her face. Daddy screamed "NO!" and lunged for the woman. The woman tried to stab Mama again, but daddy grabbed her hand. He wrestled the knife from the woman and punched her in the face. The woman fell to the ground and laid still for a minute. Daddy was holding mama telling her he was sorry but Mama wasn't saying anything. He was trying to hold Mama and was dialing his phone. I guess he was trying to call 911."

"Daddy wasn't paying attention to the woman, but after a few minutes she got up, grabbed the knife and was running toward Daddy. That's when I screamed for Daddy to look out. Daddy looked up at me with a face of horror and the woman stopped dead in her tracks. I guess my scream startled her, especially since no one had realized I was in the room. Daddy wrestled the knife from the woman again."

"When he got the knife from her he started looking for his phone. The woman calmly walked over to him and told him he wasn't going to call the police. He said why wouldn't he call the police. The woman told him because it would be her word against his. Daddy made this sound like a sarcastic laugh and told her she was crazy. The woman told him he hasn't seen crazy. She told him that the police would be very interested in the emails he sent her from his home computer email account plotting his wife's murder. Yeah, the woman laughed, you have been sending me emails for months plotting your wife's death."

"Daddy froze, then he told the woman she was lying. She looked at him and said, "Oh, you think this is a game?" Then she pulled out some papers and handed them to daddy. Daddy started reading the papers and looked up at the woman. They will never believe this came from me. They will be able to tell you set me up. The woman asked him did he want to take his chances? Daddy sat on the bed looking defeated and started to cry. The woman walked over to him and told him to man up, it was time to come home."

"Then the woman turned to me and said but first we need to take care of her. She was standing closer to me and before either of us could react she grabbed me by the neck, I couldn't breathe. I didn't see Daddy, but he must have hit her because we fell on the floor. Daddy grabbed me by my arm and pushed me behind him. He was standing in between the woman and me. He told her he would go to jail before he let her hurt me."

"I was frozen. I couldn't move. I couldn't talk. I couldn't cry, I couldn't do anything. It was like I was frozen in time. All I remember is feeling my pants were wet, I guess I had peed on myself. The woman then asked Daddy what he suggested they do with me? We will take her with us. They started to argue again about me while I was frozen in place."

"The woman finally said she had enough, they would take me with them for now but if I became a problem, a liability, I was dispensable. She went on to plot how they would make my mother's death look like an accident. She told Daddy to follow her.

Daddy told me to stay in the room and don't move. They left me standing in the middle of the room with my mother's body laid across the bed. I don't know how long I stood there before I went over to Mama."

Neecy is crying again, looking at her hands. "There was so much blood." Monica squeezes Neecy's hand and ask "Neecy, do you feel me squeezing your hand?" Neecy nods. "Do you want to continue?" Neecy nods yes. "I don't know how long they were gone, but only Daddy came back in the room. He told me to come, we had to leave now. At that point I started crying and hugging Mama laying there in a pool of blood. Daddy picked me up and said we didn't have time for this we had to go."

"Angela chimes in, when they left you in the room is when daddy must have come upstairs. He had this wild look in his eyes, a look that scared me. I had never seen him look like that before. He told me that I needed to go next door right now. He helped me put on my robe and told me to go. I remember asking him where you were and he told me now to worry about you, you were OK, just go next door like I was told. He walked me to the front door. As I was going down the steps I looked back but he had disappeared back into the house."

"I was scared because it was dark outside, I didn't know what to do. One of the neighbors was coming home and saw me standing on the sidewalk. She stopped and asked me what I was doing outside that time of night by myself. When I told her that Daddy told me to go to a neighbor's house, she looked up at our house, got this weird look on her face and told me to come with her. Once inside her house, I heard her calling the police."

"The next thing I knew we heard a loud boom. It was so loud the neighbor's house shook and then we heard sirens. I heard the neighbor's husband tell her to keep me in the house. The next thing I know a policeman was asking me questions. Shortly after that, Aunt Patty showed up and told me I was going home with her." The room is silent, all you could hear was soft sniffles. Even Monica and Miles were crying. Miles puts his arms around Neecy.

"Neecy do you know who the woman was? Would you recognize her if you saw her again? Would you be able to provide a sketch to the police?

"Yes, I would recognize her. There is no need for me to provide a sketch, I know who she is. She is the woman that I just held her memorial services. The woman I have been crying over. The woman that raised me. The woman for all these years I called my mother."

The room falls silent. No one is talking, no one knows what to say, all you can hear is breathing. Tears are streaming down Neecy's face. All of a sudden Neecy is screaming, "I watched the woman that I called Mama murder my mother! My father went along with it! All this time, I thought he loved me, cared for me, protected me, when he was only trying to save his own skin. My own father made a life with this woman, he let me call her Mama! He let me believe she was my mother! They went on living as if everything was normal."

Miles and Monica are trying to comfort Neecy while Angela and Patty are holding each other crying. Neecy drifts into her own thoughts. "How could I have forgotten all of this? I have to make sense of this. How can my mother ever forgive me for leaving her laying there, bleeding to death? I could have run and got help. I could have refused to go. I could have called 911, but I did nothing."

"Call 911! Get an ambulance here now! I was afraid this would be too much for her at one time." Neecy hears Monica saying. Patty is praying out loud, while Angela is yelling at someone that she needs an ambulance. Neecy thinks to herself, "Is she calling an ambulance for me?" Miles is screaming in Neecy's ear to hold on, but she can barely hear him over her heart beating in her ear. Neecy starts to hear her heart beating louder in her ears. The voices in the room are saying something, but she can't understand them. She feels her heart beating faster and faster, louder and louder. She can't make out what the others are saying. Her thoughts are fading, all she can remember is that she needs to breathe. "Breathe Neecy, breathe."

DISCUSSION GUIDE

1. Breathe opens with Neecy having reoccurring nightmares of being strangled. What are your thoughts as Neecy discusses her nightmare with Monica?

2. Jasper appears to be possessive and shows a potential for violence. What are your thoughts about Neecy staying with Jasper?

3. Neecy later finds out that Jasper's real name is Miles. Should Neecy stay with Miles after Finding out he has been being deceptive?

4. Discuss the nature of Neecy and Monica's relationship. Can Monica and Neecy's relationship withstand the test of time?

5. Discuss the nature of Neecy's and Alice's relationship. If Alice had not died in the fire, what would be next step for Alice and Neecy?

6. What was Alice's end goal? Discuss her motivation as the antagonist.

7. Discuss how trauma impacted Neecy's behavior.

8. Does Monica's understanding of trauma help Neecy through her crisis?

9. Discuss Miles and Monica's intent for withholding information from Neecy. Was it the best approach for Neecy?

10. Was Dale's (Neecy's father) actions selfish? Why or why not?

11. If Neecy's father were still alive, do you think they would be able to repair their relationship?

12. Does Dale deserves to be forgiven? Should Patty and Angela forgive him?

13. Discuss what Angela and Patty could have done different once Miles located Neecy.

14. Breath is the essence of life. How has reading this book changed how you think about breathing?

15. Discuss if you will do anything different as a result of what you have learned about breathing and trauma.

www.ingramcontent.com/pod-product-compliance
Lightning Source LLC
Chambersburg PA
CBHW072133270326
41931CB00010B/1752